全国医药中等职业教育药学类"十四五"规划教材（第三轮）

供医药卫生类专业使用

医药英语 （第3版）

主　编　常光萍　甘　霞

主　审　Elizabeth H. M. Jones

副主编　田　莉　张　坤　王小玲

编　者　（以姓氏笔画为序）

　　　　王小玲（天水市卫生学校）

　　　　方梦婕（江西省医药学校）

　　　　甘　霞（四川省食品药品学校）

　　　　田　莉（上海市医药学校）

　　　　沈　柳（上海市医药学校）

　　　　张　坤（广州市医药职业学校）

　　　　陈　林（上海市医药学校）

　　　　陈兰英（湛江中医学校）

　　　　罗　凡（上海市医药学校）

　　　　常光萍（上海市医药学校）

　　　　蔡　莉（上海市医药学校）

U0286174

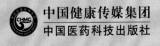

中国健康传媒集团

中国医药科技出版社

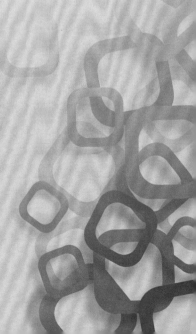

内 容 提 要

　　本教材是全国医药中等职业教育药学类"十四五"规划教材（第三轮）之一，根据医药英语教学大纲的基本要求和课程特点编写而成。本书以人体八大系统的常见疾病为主题，选择了哮喘、感冒与咳嗽、心绞痛、糖尿病、酗酒、抑郁症及艾滋病等16种常见疾病，形成了16个单元的主题。本书具有科学性、趣味性及实用性等特点，适用于有初级英语语言基础的药学、护理、制药技术及医学技术等专业的医药职业院校学生，也适合在医药健康行业从事涉外业务的医药生产、销售及医护人员使用。

图书在版编目（CIP）数据

　　医药英语/常光萍，甘霞主编. —3 版. —北京：中国医药科技出版社，2020. 12
　　全国医药中等职业教育药学类"十四五"规划教材. 第三轮
　　ISBN 978 – 7 – 5214 – 2129 – 3

　　I. ①医… II. ①常… ②甘… III. ①医药学 – 英语 – 中等专业学校 – 教材 IV. ①R

　　中国版本图书馆 CIP 数据核字（2020）第 236580 号

美术编辑　陈君杞
版式设计　友全图文

出版　**中国健康传媒集团** | 中国医药科技出版社
地址　北京市海淀区文慧园北路甲 22 号
邮编　100082
电话　发行：010 – 62227427　邮购：010 – 62236938
网址　www. cmstp. com
规格　787mm×1092mm $^{1}/_{16}$
印张　14 $^{3}/_{4}$
字数　283 千字
初版　2011 年 5 月第 1 版
版次　2020 年 12 月第 3 版
印次　2023 年 8 月第 3 次印刷
印刷　三河市万龙印装有限公司
经销　全国各地新华书店
书号　ISBN 978 – 7 – 5214 – 2129 – 3
定价　**58. 00 元**

获取新书信息、投稿、为图书纠错，请扫码联系我们。

出版说明

2011 年，中国医药科技出版社根据教育部《中等职业教育改革创新行动计划（2010—2012 年）》精神，组织编写出版了"全国医药中等职业教育药学类专业规划教材"；2016 年，根据教育部 2014 年颁发的《中等职业学校专业教学标准（试行）》等文件精神，修订出版了第二轮规划教材"全国医药中等职业教育药学类'十三五'规划教材"，受到广大医药卫生类中等职业院校师生的欢迎。为了进一步提升教材质量，紧跟职教改革形势，根据教育部颁发的《国家职业教育改革实施方案》（国发〔2019〕4 号）、《中等职业学校专业教学标准（试行）》（教职成厅函〔2014〕48 号）精神，中国医药科技出版社有限公司经过广泛征求各有关院校及专家的意见，于 2020 年 3 月正式启动了第三轮教材的编写工作。在教育部、国家药品监督管理局的领导和指导下，在本套教材建设指导委员会专家的指导和顶层设计下，中国医药科技出版社有限公司组织全国 60 余所院校 300 余名教学经验丰富的专家、教师精心编撰了"全国医药中等职业教育药学类'十四五'规划教材（第三轮）"，该套教材付梓出版。

本套教材共计 42 种，全部配套"医药大学堂"在线学习平台。主要供全国医药卫生中等职业院校药学类专业教学使用，也可供医药卫生行业从业人员继续教育和培训使用。

本套教材定位清晰，特点鲜明，主要体现如下几个方面。

1. 立足教改，适应发展

为了适应职业教育教学改革需要，教材注重以真实生产项目、典型工作任务为载体组织教学单元。遵循职业教育规律和技术技能型人才成长规律，体现中职药学人才培养的特点，着力提高药学类专业学生的实践操作能力。以学生的全面素质培养和产业对人才的要求为教学目标，按职业教育"需求驱动"型课程建构的过程，进行任务分析。坚持理论知识"必需、够用"为度。强调教材的针对性、实用性、条理性和先进性，既注重对学生基本技能的培养，又适当拓展知识面，实现职业教育与终身学习的对接，为学生后续发展奠定必要的基础。

2. 强化技能，对接岗位

教材要体现中等职业教育的属性，使学生掌握一定的技能以适应岗位的需要，具有一定的理论知识基础和可持续发展的能力。理论知识把握有度，既要给学生学习和掌握技能奠定必要的、足够的理论基础，也不要过分强调理论知识的系统性和完整性；

注重技能结合理论知识，建设理论－实践一体化教材。

3. 优化模块，易教易学

设计生动、活泼的教学模块，在保持教材主体框架的基础上，通过模块设计增加教材的信息量和可读性、趣味性。例如通过引入实际案例以及岗位情景模拟，使教材内容更贴近岗位，让学生了解实际岗位的知识与技能要求，做到学以致用；"请你想一想"模块，便于师生教学的互动；"你知道吗"模块适当介绍新技术、新设备以及科技发展新趋势、行业职业资格考试与现代职业发展相关知识，为学生后续发展奠定必要的基础。

4. 产教融合，优化团队

现代职业教育倡导职业性、实践性和开放性，职业教育必须校企合作、工学结合、学作融合。专业技能课教材，鼓励吸纳1～2位具有丰富实践经验的企业人员参与编写，确保工作岗位上的先进技术和实际应用融入教材内容，更加体现职业教育的职业性、实践性和开放性。

5. 多媒融合，数字增值

为适应现代化教学模式需要，本套教材搭载"医药大学堂"在线学习平台，配套以纸质教材为基础的多样化数字教学资源（如课程PPT、习题库、微课等），使教材内容更加生动化、形象化、立体化。此外，平台尚有数据分析、教学诊断等功能，可为教学研究与管理提供技术和数据支撑。

编写出版本套高质量教材，得到了全国各相关院校领导与编者的大力支持，在此一并表示衷心感谢。出版发行本套教材，希望得到广大师生的欢迎，并在教学中积极使用和提出宝贵意见，以便修订完善，共同打造精品教材，为促进我国中等职业教育医药类专业教学改革和人才培养作出积极贡献。

全国医药中等职业教育药学类"十四五"规划教材(第三轮)

◦ 建设指导委员会名单 ◦

主 任 委 员 　张耀华　中国药师协会

副主任委员 （以姓氏笔画为序）

刘运福	辽宁医药职业学院	阳　欢	江西省医药学校
孙师家	广东省食品药品职业技术学校	李　刚	亳州中药科技学校
李　冰	淄博市技师学院	李榆梅	天津药科中等专业学校
沈雁平	淮南职业教育中心	宋向前	天水市卫生学校
张雪昀	湖南食品药品职业学院	张福莹	潍坊弘景中医药学校
张橡楠	河南医药健康技师学院	周　琦	广西中医药大学附设中医学校
贾　强	山东药品食品职业学院	倪　汀	江苏省常州技师学院
蒋忠元	上海市医药学校	程　敏	四川省食品药品学校
靳柯娟	安徽阜阳技师学院	薛亚明	北京实验职业学校

委员 （以姓氏笔画为序）

丁冬梅	广东省食品药品职业技术学校	马　昕	本溪市化学工业学校
王小佳	揭阳市卫生学校	王金鹏	四川省食品药品学校
王桂梅	山东药品食品职业学院	厉　欢	河南医药健康技师学院
石　磊	江西省医药学校	卢延颖	本溪市化学工业学校
卢楚霞	广东省新兴中药学校	田　洋	本溪市化学工业学校
冯建华	四川省食品药品学校	巩海涛	山东药品食品职业学院
吕　慎	上海市医药学校	刘　波	上海市医药学校
刘开林	四川省食品药品学校	刘长久	四川省食品药品学校
刘巧元	湖南食品药品职业学院	刘桂丽	江苏省常州技师学院
许瑞林	江苏省常州技师学院	孙　晓	山东药品食品职业学院

苏兰宜	江西省医药学校	杨永庆	天水市卫生学校
李　芳	珠海市卫生学校	李应军	四川省食品药品学校
李桂兰	江西省医药学校	李桂荣	山东药品食品职业学院
李承革	四川省食品药品学校	何　红	江西省医药学校
张　玲	山东药品食品职业学院	张一帆	山东药品食品职业学院
张小明	四川省食品药品学校	陈　静	江西省医药学校
林　勇	江西省医药学校	林　楠	上海市医药学校
欧阳小青	广东省食品药品职业技术学校	欧绍淑	广东省湛江卫生学校
尚金燕	山东药品食品职业学院	罗　翀	湖南食品药品职业学院
罗玲英	江西省医药学校	周　容	四川省食品药品学校
郑小吉	广东省江门中医药学校	柯宇新	广东省食品药品职业技术学校
赵　磊	四川省食品药品学校	赵珍东	广东省食品药品职业技术学校
秦胜红	四川省食品药品学校	贾效彬	亳州中药科技学校
夏玉玲	四川省食品药品学校	高　娟	山东药品食品职业学院
高丽丽	江西省医药学校	郭常文	四川省食品药品学校
黄　瀚	湖南食品药品职业学院	常光萍	上海市医药学校
崔　艳	上海市医药学校	董树裔	上海市医药学校
鲍　娜	湖南食品药品职业学院		

全国医药中等职业教育药学类"十四五"规划教材（第三轮）

———◦ 评审委员会名单 ◦———

数字化教材编委会

主　编　常光萍　甘　霞
主　审　Elizabeth H. M. Jones
副主编　田　莉　张　坤　王小玲
编　者　（以姓氏笔画为序）
　　　　王小玲（天水市卫生学校）
　　　　方梦婕（江西省医药学校）
　　　　甘　霞（四川省食品药品学校）
　　　　田　莉（上海市医药学校）
　　　　沈　柳（上海市医药学校）
　　　　张　坤（广州市医药职业学校）
　　　　陈　林（上海市医药学校）
　　　　陈兰英（湛江中医学校）
　　　　罗　凡（上海市医药学校）
　　　　常光萍（上海市医药学校）
　　　　蔡　莉（上海市医药学校）

近年来，我国生物医药及大健康产业发展迅猛，并伴随着日益繁荣的国际交往与合作。为了满足医药产业的国际化发展对技术技能人才的特定需求，同时更好地服务学生的职业生涯发展，我们编写了《医药英语》教材，用来培养学生在职场环境下运用英语的基本能力，同时提高他们的综合文化素养和跨文化交际水平。

本教材围绕人体运动系统、循环系统、呼吸系统、消化系统、泌尿系统、生殖系统、神经系统和内分泌系统中的常见问题，以哮喘、感冒与咳嗽、心绞痛、糖尿病、酗酒、抑郁症及艾滋病等16种常见病症为各单元的主题。选材过程中密切关注医学和药学的最新进展，尤其是听力部分的内容涉及到国内外的先进医药技术及发展动态。

教材内容选取和结构安排充分考虑医药职业院校学生的学习特点及语言能力。在内容上，每个单元的各板块均围绕单元主题即一种常见疾病进行编写，在确保其科学性的同时突出趣味性及实用性，使学习者在具有生活体验或背景知识的情境下学习医药类专业的英文表达，逐步提升其英语语言素养。在结构上，每单元由导入、会话、阅读、词汇、练习及听力六部分组成。具体来讲，导入部分采用有趣的图片或常识测试等方式来激发学生学习兴趣，进而创设切题的学习环境；会话部分设定为围绕一个健康问题由医生与患者、药剂师（员）与患者、朋友或者家人间的交流，内容较为生活化，相对简单易懂，语言也更口语化、实用化；阅读部分为长度约500个单词的文章，选取了较为通俗易懂的近科普类文章，避免学术性专业文献的生涩、枯燥，文后附有文中出现的专业词汇以及重要的词汇和句型讲解，以便学生有方向、有目的地掌握医药学环境中的英语表达；在形式上采用了更活泼的分块排版，避免阅读时出现疲劳感；练习的编写凸显了单元知识点的巩固，针对性强，在做练习中强化、升华；听力部分选取了与单元主题密切相关的医药专业人士对话、讲座或采访，为学习者提供真实的语言背景，使其更好地了解相关内容，并拓展专业视野。

本教材为书网融合教材，即纸质教材有机融合电子教材、教学配套资源（PPT、微课、语音）、题库系统、数字化教学服务等，使教学资源更加多样，便于学生更好地学习、使用。

　　本教材由长期从事中外合作办学项目管理及教学工作的常光萍、长期从事职业学校英语教学实践与研究的甘霞任主编，田莉、张坤及王小玲任副主编，加拿大籍资深英语教育专家 Elizabeth H. M. Jones 女士主审。编写人员还有蔡莉、沈柳、罗凡、陈林、方梦婕及陈兰英等。贾俊负责书中插图的绘制及拍摄，指导学生屡次获得全国职业院校职业英语技能大赛一等奖的马增彩老师及有医药企业工作经历和海外留学背景的戴婧老师提出了许多宝贵意见，本教材的数字化资源还采用了朱柳柳老师录制的部分微课，在此一并表示感谢。由于受编者学识所限，书中难免存在疏漏与不足，恳请读者批评指正。

编者

2020 年 10 月

OBJECTIVES

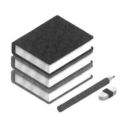

When you have completed Unit 1, you will be able to

⊙ understand and identify professional terms related to asthma.

⊙ communicate with the chemist about the asthma drug properly.

⊙ skim the passage for main idea.

⊙ describe the symptoms, the causes and the control of asthma.

⊙ obtain information about asthma by listening to the lecture.

⊙ master the uses of *it*.

LEAD IN

"Is Asthma Draining the Life out of You?"

Are you tired of suffering from…

⊙ shortness of breath or losing your breath easily.

⊙ frequent cough, especially at night.

⊙ feeling very tired or weak all the time.

⊙ embarrassing wheezing or coughing easily.

⊙ feeling tired, easily upset, grouchy, suffocated, or moody.

⊙ constant decreases or changes in your lung function.

⊙ signs of a cold or allergies.

⊙ sneezing, runny nose, cough, nasal congestion, sore throat, and headache.

⊙ chest tightness, pain, or pressure.

⊙ trouble sleeping or insomnia.

⊙ asthma attacks.

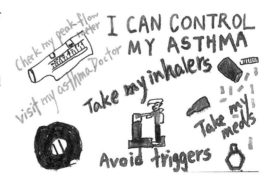

Which of the above symptoms are about asthma?

📑 CONVERSATION

会话

Asthma

It is February. A young man enters the drugstore.

Linda：Hello! Welcome!

Youngman：I'm looking for "Spiropent".

Linda：For yourself?

Youngman：Yes. I'm asthmatic, and here's my prescription.

Linda：Thank you, I'll just enter this in our computer and check our stock.

Youngman：Thanks. This is my first time. Would you give me some information?

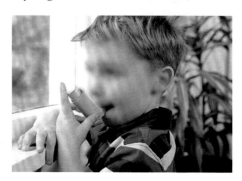

Linda：Of course, that's our job. Here is your medication, and in the box are some clear instructions. Doctors commonly prescribe this drug because it's so effective. Now, as you probably know, asthma is very common and affects the respiratory system. There is a high incidence during spring and winter.

Young man：For sure!

Linda：You should also watch your diet and lifestyle.

Youngman：Oh! I didn't know that.

Linda：Yes! Don't overdo it with sweet and greasy junk food, or even spicy food. And you should get in the habit of moderate, regular exercise.

Young man：Well, I guess it's worth to be healthy. Thanks for your time.

Linda：That's what we're here for, please call if you have any questions or complications or contact your doctor.

Activity

Suppose your close friend has asthma. What should he/she pay attention to?

📑 READING

Asthma

Pre – reading

What is asthma?

What are the symptoms?

What triggers an asthma attack?

How can asthma be managed?

While – reading

What Is Asthma? [e] 微课 1

Asthma is a chronic disease characterized by recurrent attacks of breathlessness and wheezing, which vary in severity and frequency from person to person.[1]

Symptoms may occur several times in a day or week in affected individuals, and for some people become worse during physical activity or at night.

An Asthma Attack [e] 微课 2

During an asthma attack, the lining of the bronchial tubes swells, causing the airways to narrow and reducing the flow of air into and out of the lungs. Recurrent asthma symptoms frequently cause sleeplessness, daytime fatigue, reduced activity levels and school and work absenteeism. Asthma has a relatively low fatality rate compared to other chronic diseases.

What Triggers an Asthma Attack? [e] 微课 3

Some causes and triggers are common to all people with asthma, and some are more individual. Although the fundamental causes of asthma are not completely understood, the strongest risk factors for developing asthma are inhaled asthma triggers. These include:

⊙ indoor allergens (for example house dust mites in bedding, carpets and stuffed furniture, pollution and pet dander)

⊙ outdoor allergens (such as pollens and moulds)

⊙ tobacco smoke

⊙ chemical irritants in the workplace

⊙ air pollution

Other Triggers

Other triggers can include cold air, extreme emotional arousal such as anger or fear, and physical exercise. In some people, asthma can even be triggered by certain medications,[2] such as aspirin and other non-steroid anti-inflammatory drugs, and beta-blockers (which are used to treat high blood pressure, heart conditions and migraine). Urbanization has also been associated with an increase in asthma; however the exact nature of this relationship is unclear.

Management of Asthma

According to WHO estimates, 235 million people suffer from asthma globally. Although asthma cannot be cured,[2] appropriate management can control the disorder and enable people to enjoy good quality of life. In addition, some children with milder forms of asthma outgrow their symptoms with age.

Short-term medications are used to relieve symptoms.[2] People with persistent symptoms must take long-term medication daily to control the underlying inflammation and prevent symptoms and exacerbations.

Medication is not the only way to control asthma. It is also important to avoid asthma triggers-stimuli that irritate and inflame the airways.[3] With medical support, each asthma patient must learn what triggers he or she should avoid.

Although asthma does not kill on the scale of chronic obstructive pulmonary disease (COPD) or other chronic diseases, failure to use appropriate medications or to adhere to treatment can lead to death.

WHO recognizes that asthma is of major public health significance. The organization plays a role in coordinating international efforts against the disease. The aim of its strategy is to support Member States in their efforts to reduce the disability and premature death related to asthma.

Notes

1. Asthma is a chronic disease characterized by recurrent attacks of breathlessness and wheezing, which vary in severity and frequency from person to person.

此句为 which 引导的非限制性定语从句。后半句起补充说明作用，缺少也不会影响全句的理解，在非限定性定语从句的前面往往有逗号隔开，如若将非限定性定语从句放在句子中间，其前后都需要用逗号隔开。

如：In the presence of so many people he was a little tense, which was understandable.

在那么多人面前他有点紧张，这是可以理解的。

He may have acute appendicitis, in which case he will have to be operated on.

他可能得了急性盲肠炎，如果是这样，他就得动手术。

When deeply absorbed in work, which he often was, he would forget all about eating and sleeping.

他经常聚精会神地工作，这时他会废寝忘食。

2. In some people, asthma can even be triggered by certain medications.

Although asthma cannot be cured, appropriate management can control the disorder and enable people to enjoy a good quality of life.

Short-term medications are used to relieve symptoms.

上述三句都是被动语态的句子。被动语态是动词的一种特殊形式，一般说来，只有需要动作对象的及物动词才有被动语态。汉语往往用"被""受""给"等词来表示被动意义。被动语态由"助动词 be + 及物动词的过去分词"构成。人称、数和时态的变化是通过 be 的变化表现出来的。

3. It is also important to avoid asthma triggers-stimuli that irritate and inflame the airways.

该句中 it 是形式主语，真正的主语是 to avoid asthma triggers-stimuli that irritate and inflame the airways.

当代英语中，通常用 it 做形式主语，将不定式和动名词置于谓语后面，特别是主语较长时，或在一些习惯用法中。

It isn't right to speak ill of someone behind his back.

在别人背后说坏话是不对的。

It is not an easy thing to master a foreign language.

掌握一门外语不是件容易的事。

It is my duty to care for that patient.

照料那位病人是我的职责。

Glossary

Word	English definition	Example
recurrent *adj.*	occurring again and again	Evidence shows that fluid intake is very effective in staving off recurrent kidney stone attacks
absenteeism *n.*	habitual missed time from work	His boss discharged him for habitual absenteeism
trigger *n.*	an act that sets in motion some course of events	A desire to earn high marks triggered habits of diligent study
inhale *v.*	drawair deeply into the lungs by breathing	Researchers spray the vaccine up an animal's nose and they breathe it out where it remains airborne and is inhaled by animals within two metres of them
allergen *n.*	any substance that can cause an allergy, a potentially dangerous physical reaction, such as sneezing, skin rash, swelling	Regarding elimination diets, please see my answer above regarding food allergens and migraine
relieve *v.*	provide physical respite, as from pain	The aspirin relieved her headache within about fifteen minutes

Word	English definition	Chinese definition
asthma *n.*	respiratory disorder characterized by wheezing; usually of allergic origin	哮喘
wheezing *adj.*	relating to breathing with a whistling sound	气喘
bronchial *adj.*	relating to or associated with the bronchi, small breathing tubes in the lungs	支气管的
mite *n.*	any of numerous very small to minute arachnids often infesting animals or plants or stored foods	小虫

Word	English definition	Chinese definition
dander *n.*	small scales from animal skins or hair or bird feathers that can cause allergic reactions in some people	头皮屑
pollen *n.*	the fine spores that contain male gametes and that are borne by an anther in a flowering plant	［植］花粉
mould *n.*	a fungus that produces a superficial growth on various kinds of damp or decaying organic matter	霉菌
steroid *n.*	any of several fat-soluble organic compounds having as a basis 17 carbon atoms in four rings；many have important physiological effects	类固醇

Post – reading

A1. Scan the text and complete the sentence.

1. During an asthma attack，the lining of the ＿＿＿＿＿ ＿＿＿＿＿ swells，causing the airways to ＿＿＿＿＿ and thereby reducing the flow of air into and out of the lungs.

2. Asthma has a relatively low ＿＿＿＿＿ ＿＿＿＿＿ compared to other chronic diseases.

3. The strongest risk factors for developing asthma are ＿＿＿＿＿ ＿＿＿＿＿ ＿＿＿＿＿ .

4. Other triggers can include ＿＿＿＿＿ ＿＿＿＿＿，extreme emotional arousal such as anger or fear，and physical exercise.

5. In some people，asthma can even be triggered by ＿＿＿＿＿ ＿＿＿＿＿ .

6. Short-term medications are used to ＿＿＿＿＿ ＿＿＿＿＿ .

A2. Decide whether the following sentences are true or false. Write T for true and F for false.

1. Asthma is an acute disease characterized by recurrent attacks of breathlessness and wheezing. ＿＿＿＿＿

2. During an asthma attack，the lining of the bronchial tubes swells. ＿＿＿＿＿

3. Asthma has a relatively high fatality rate compared to other chronic diseases. ＿＿＿＿＿

4. Some causes and triggers are common to all people with asthma，and some are more individual. ＿＿＿＿＿

5. An inhaled asthma trigger is not the main problem for developing asthma. _____

6. In some people, asthma can even be triggered by certain medications. _____

B1. Choose the appropriate words and fill in the blanks with their correct forms.

| relieve | persistent | inflammatory | outgrow |
| exacerbations | beta-blocker | stimuli | chronic |

1. An allergy is an _____ response of the immune system to substances that would not cause activation of the immune system in persons who are not allergic.

2. The next day, they saw the pictures again, but half were given the drug propranolol, a _____ commonly used to treat heart disease.

3. You had better open your mouth to _____ the pressure on your eardrums.

4. _____ damage or inadequate healing may lead to chronic lameness.

5. Considering the high prevalence of asthma, especially among young people, we suggest that this type of trigger be considered in the assessment of asthma _____ .

6. The illness frequently coexists with other _____ diseases.

7. Our muscles have to be trained to react in certain ways to certain _____ .

8. These mutant plants eventually _____ the infection.

B2. Match the following words with their English meaning.

Word	Meaning
1) inflammatory	a. provide physical relief, as from pain
2) migraine	b. never-ceasing
3) relieve	c. any stimulating information or event; acts to arouse action
4) persistent	d. characterized or caused by inflammation
5) exacerbation	e. a severe recurring vascular headache; occurs more frequently in women than men
6) stimulus	f. action that makes a problem or a disease (or its symptoms) worse

B3. Fill in the blanks with the words in the text. The first letter is given to you.

1. The rabbit is c _____ by its long ears.

2. Aspirin can ulcerate the stomach l _____ .

3. For much of his life he suffered from r _____ bouts of depression.

4. They think his mother's illness is acute rather than c _____ .

5. Apart from clothes and b _____ , I have nothing.

6. Every case he had was already s _____ with clothes.

C1. Translate the following sentences into Chinese.

1. Recurrent asthma symptoms frequently cause sleeplessness, daytime fatigue, reduced

activity levels and school and work absenteeism.

2. Other triggers can include cold air, extreme emotional arousal such as anger or fear, and physical exercise.

3. Urbanization has also been associated with an increase in asthma, however the exact nature of this relationship is unclear.

4. Although asthma cannot be cured, appropriate management can control the disorder and enable people to enjoy good quality of life.

5. In addition, some children with milder forms of asthma outgrow their symptoms with age.

6. People with persistent symptoms must take long-term medication daily to control the underlying inflammation and prevent symptoms and exacerbations.

C2. Choose the best answer for the following exercise.

1. It takes me 30 minutes _____ to school by bike every day.

    A. going   B. to go   C. goes   D. go

2. It's not easy _____ us _____ a foreign language.

    A. for; learning   B. of; learning   C. of; to learn   D. for; to learn

3. Children find _____ interesting to play computer games.

    A. that   B. which   C. it   D. he

4. Do you think it important _____ computer well?

    A. play   B. plays   C. to play   D. playing

5. Is _____ necessary to complete the design before national day?

    A. this   B. that   C. it   D. he

C3. Translate the following sentences into English.

1. 小女孩慢慢长大后就不再怕宠物了。(outgrow)

2. 事实证明，微笑和大笑能够缓解焦虑和压力。(relieve)

3. 吸烟导致每年有 1 万人死于慢性肺病。(chronic)

4. 压力可能会成为引发这些疾病的原因。(trigger)

5. 牙医可能会决定拔掉那颗牙，以免反复发作。(recurrent)

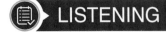 **LISTENING**

听力

Fill in the blanks according to what you hear.

WHAT CAUSES ASTHMA?

People with asthma have inflamed airways that are supersensitive to things which do not bother other people. These things are called "triggers." Although asthma "triggers" vary from person to person, some of the most common include:

⊙ ubstances/allergens such as dust mites, pollens, moulds, _____ dander, and even cockroaches and their _____ .

⊙ irritants in the air, including _____ from cigarettes, _____ fires or charcoal grills. Also, strong _____ or odors like household sprays, paint, petrol (gasoline), perfume, and scented _____ .

⊙ respiratory infections such as _____ , flu, sore throats, and sinus _____ . These are the most common asthma triggers in children.

⊙ exercise and other activities that make you breathe harder.

⊙ _____ such as dry wind, cold air, or _____ changes in weather.

书网融合……

微课1

微课2

微课3

自测题

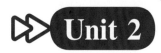 **Unit 2** **Cold and Cough**

PPT

 OBJECTIVES

When you have completed Unit 2, you will be able to

⊙ understand and identify professional terms related to cold and cough.

⊙ communicate with the chemist about some typical symptoms properly.

⊙ skim the passage for main idea.

⊙ describe the symptoms, the causes and the control of abuse of cold and cough remedies.

⊙ obtain information about cold and cough by listening to the lecture.

⊙ master the uses of past participles.

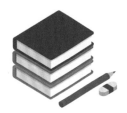

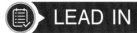 **LEAD IN**

Natural Cold and Flu Remedies

It's no wonder natural cold and flu remedies are popular — modern medicine has yet to offer a cure for these age-old ailments. While some medications can prevent and shorten the flu's duration, some medications only offer temporary relief of symptoms. Many natural remedies provide temporary relief as well, and a few may actually help you get better. Here are some remedies.

Match the following pictures with the words

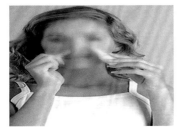
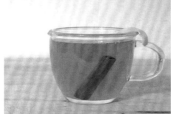
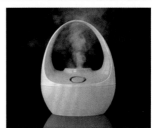

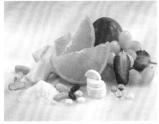
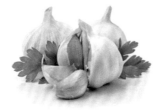
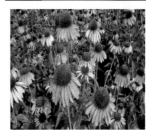

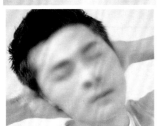
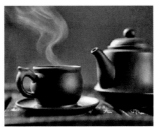
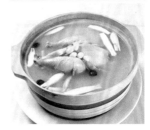

1. Echinacea   2. Vitamin C   3. Chicken Soup   4. Hot Tea   5. Garlic   6. Humidifier

7. Saline Drops   8. Nasal Strips   9. Hot Toddy

CONVERSATION

Where is the Cough Medicine?

It's early evening on Wednesday. A middle-aged woman enters the drugstore.

John: Good evening, madam. Can I help you?

Woman: Good evening. I want to buy some cough medicine.

John: Is it for you?

Woman: No, it's for my husband.

John: What are his symptoms?

Woman: He has been coughing up phlegm. Moreover he

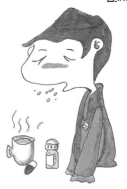

Cough

has a fever, a headache, a stuffy nose and aching limbs.

John: Is the phlegm yellow or white?

Woman: Thin and white.

John: Has he ever had pulmonary tuberculosis?

Woman: No, he hasn't.

John: Then, I recommend you to buy a bottle of *Sanshedan Chuanbeilu* oral solution for him. It's cheap and the effect is good.

Woman: OK, I'd like to take it. Can you tell me how to use it?

John: Yes, Please take ten or twenty milliliters each time, three times a day after meals. Please go to see a doctor if there's no effect after three days.

Woman: I'll remember all that. Thanks a lot.

John: You can always read the label or give us a call. I hope your husband feels better soon.

Activity

Practice the dialogue and make adialogue of your own.

Situation: Suppose that your close friend had a bad fever, and you want to show your concern.

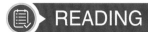 **READING**

Cough and Cold Medicine Abuse

Pre – reading

Why do kids abuse cough and cold remedies?

What's the major difference between current abuse of cough and cold medicines and that in years past?

What happens when teens abuse DXM?

How can we prevent teens from abusing over-the-counter medicines?

While – reading

Chugging cough medicine for an instant high isn't a new practice for teens[1] who have raided the medicine cabinet for a quick, cheap, and legal high for decades. And unfortunately, this dangerous, potentially deadly practice still goes on.

So it's important for parents to understand the risks and know how to prevent their kids from intentionally overdosing on cough and cold medicine.

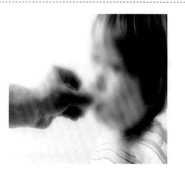

Why Do Kids Abuse Cough and Cold Remedies?

Before the U. S. Food and Drug Administration (FDA) replaced the narcotic codeine with dextromethorphan as an over-the-counter (OTC) cough suppressant in the 1970s, teens were simply guzzling down cough syrup for a quick buzz.

Over the years, teens discovered that they still could get high by taking large doses of any OTC medicine containing dextromethorphan (also called DXM).

Medicines containing dextromethorphan are easy to find, affordable for cash-strapped teens, and perfectly legal. Getting access to the dangerous drug is often as easy as walking into the local drugstore with a few dollars or raiding the family medicine cabinet. And because it's found in over-the-counter medicines, many teens naively assume that DXM can't be dangerous.

Then and Now

DXM abuse is common, according to recent studies, and easy access to OTC medications in stores and over the Internet probably contributes to this.

The major difference between current abuse of cough and cold medicines and that in years past is that teens now use the Internet to not only buy DXM in pure powder form, but also to learn how to abuse it. Because drinking large volumes of cough syrup causes vomiting, the drug is being extracted from cough syrups and sold on the Internet in a tablet that can be swallowed or a powder that can be snorted. Online dosing calculators even teach abusers how much they'll need to take for their weight to get high.

One way teens get their DXM fixes is by taking "Triple-C"— Coricidin HBP Cough and Cold — which contains 30mg of DXM in little red tablets. Users taking large volumes of Triple-C run additional health risks because it contains an antihistamine as well.

The list of other ingredients-decongestants, expectorants, and pain relievers-contained in other Coricidin products and OTC cough and cold preparations compound the risks associated with DXM and could lead to a serious drug overdose.

What Happens When Teens Abuse DXM?

Although DXM can be safely taken in 15 to 30 milligram doses to suppress a cough, abusers tend to consume as much as 360 milligrams or more. Taking mass quantities of products containing DXM can cause hallucinations, loss of motor control, and "out-of-body" sensations.

Other possible side effects of DXM abuse include: confusion, impaired judgment, blurred vision, dizziness, excessive sweating, slurred speech, nausea, vomiting, abdominal pain, irregular heartbeat, high blood pressure, headache, numbness of fingers and toes, facial redness, dry and itchy skin, loss of consciousness, brain damage, and even death.

When consumed in large quantities, DXM can also cause hyperthermia, or high fever. This is a real concern for teens who take DXM while in a hot environment or while exerting themselves at a rave or dance club, where DXM is often sold and passed off as similar-looking drugs like PCP. And the situation becomes even more dangerous if these substances are used with alcohol or another drug.

Being on the Lookout

You can help prevent your teen from abusing over-the-counter medicines. Here's how:

⊙ lock your medicine cabinet or keep those OTC medicines that could potentially be abused in a less accessible place.

⊙ avoid stockpiling OTC medicines. Having too many at your teen's disposal could make abusing them more tempting.

⊙ keep track of how much is in each bottle or container in your medicine cabinet.

⊙ keep an eye out not only for traditional-looking cough and cold remedies in your teen's room, but also strange-looking tablets (DXM is often sold on the Internet and on the street in its pure form in various shapes and colors).

⊙ watch out for the possible warning signs of DXM abuse.

⊙ monitor your teen's Internet use. Be on the lookout for suspicious websites and emails that seem to be promoting the abuse of DXM or other drugs, both legal and illegal.

Above all, talk to your kids about drug abuse and explain that even though taking lots of a cough or cold medicine seems harmless, it's not. Even when it comes from the family medicine cabinet or the corner drugstore, when taken in large amounts DXM is a drug that can be just as deadly as any sold on a seedy street corner. [2] And even if you don't think your teens are doing it, chances are they know others who are.

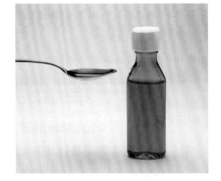

Notes

1. Chugging cough medicine for an instant high isn't a new practice for teens.

此句是动名词短语作为主语。当动名词或动名词短语作主语时，放在句首。

e. g. Learning a foreign language is very useful to everyone.

　　Reading in bed is bad for your eyes.

当动名词及其短语放在行为动词介词后，作宾语。

e. g. Have you finished doing your homework ?

　　He is not good at making friends.

注意事项：

（1）动名词作主语表单数概念，谓语动词用单数形式。

e. g. Walking after supper is good for your health.

（2）动名词作动词宾语，往往是一些固定搭配，常跟动名词作宾语的动词有：finish，enjoy，mind，practice，deny，consider，suggest，admit，put off，insist on 等。

（3）动名词的复合结构（物主代词、名词所有格是动名词逻辑上的主语、动名词是其逻辑上的谓语）作主语和宾语。

①动名词复合结构作主语

e. g. Your coming made us happy.

　　Your father's cooking is very good.

②动名词的复合结构作宾语

e. g. Do you mind my smoking?

　　My friend insisted on my staying here.

2. Even when it comes from the family medicine cabinet or the corner drugstore, when taken in large amounts DXM is a drug that can be just as deadly as any sold on a seedy street corner.

此句中 when taken in large amounts，是过去分词短语作为时间状语。过去分词用作状语，表示时间、原因、条件、让步、方式、伴随等，多数情况下相当于一个省略了连词、主语和动词 be 的状语从句。其逻辑主语一般和句子的主语一致，在大多数情况下有被动的含义。过去分词相当于副词作状语，通常表示时间、原因、条件、或伴随情况等。作状语的过去分词通常与句子的主语存在着被动关系，它所表示的动作通常和谓语动词属于同一时间范畴，也可表示先于谓语动词发生的动作。有时，为了强调先发生的动作，也可用 having been。动词过去分词形式作状语，有时前面带有连词，是状语从句的省略结构，其中省去了从句的主语和 be 动词，通常该主语与主句相同。

Glossary

Word	English definition	Example
chug *v.*	to drink alcohol really fast without breathing	The loser of a game is required to chug a beer
raid *v.*	to rummage through something, with the intent to find a specific item	She made her way to the kitchen to raid the fridge
intentionally *adv.*	with premeditation; in a deliberate manner.	The student intentionally lost her homework paper, hoping the teacher would forget about giving her another one
suppressant *n.*	a drug that curbs or reduces a physical urge such as appetite, itching or coughing	When the woman coughed so much she could not sleep, she asked her doctor for a cough suppressant medication
guzzle *v.*	drinkor eat greedily or as if with great thirst	Guzzling pizza and beer is not only unmannerly but unhealthy because the calories add up too quickly
vomit *v.*	eject the contents of the stomach through the mouth	She has been vomiting all night
impaired *adj.*	diminished in strength, quality, or utility	Too much reading has impaired his vision
blurred *adj.*	indistinct or hazy in outline	As the bullet train gained speed, the landscape blurred because it was too fast to see clearly
slurred *adj.*	spoken as if with a thick tongue	He slurred his English. No man could understand him
rave *n.*	a dance party that lasts all night and electronically synthesized music is played	The Saturday rave craze seems to be on the way out
seedy *adj.*	shabby and untidy	People living in the seedy city have bad lives

Word	English definition	Chinese definition
narcotic *adj.*	of or relating to a powerful mind-altering substance, possibly illegal	麻醉的；有麻醉作用的
dextromethorphan *n.*	a kind of cough medicine	右美沙芬（镇咳药）
snort *n.*	inhale through the nose	吸食（毒品）
coricidin *n.*	an antihistamine	柯利西锭（抗感冒药）
antihistamine *n.*	a medicine used to treat allergies and hypersensitive reactions and colds	抗组胺药
hallucinations *n.*	illusory perception	［心理］幻觉

Post – reading

A1. Scan the text and complete the sentence

1. Drinking large volumes of cough syrup causes _____ .

2. DXM can be safely taken in _____ doses to suppress a cough.

3. Lock your medicine cabinet or keep those OTC medicines that could potentially be abused in a less _____ place.

4. Avoid stockpiling OTC medicines. Having too many at your teen's _____ could make abusing them more tempting.

5. Keep _____ of how much is in each bottle or container in your medicine cabi-

net.

6. Be on the lookout for _____ websites and emails that seem to be promoting the abuse of DXM or other drugs, both legal and illegal.

A2. Translate the following sentences into Chinese

1. Chugging cough medicine for an instant high isn't a new practice for teens.

2. It's important for parents to understand the risks and know how to prevent their kids from intentionally overdosing on cough and cold medicine.

3. Medicines containing dextromethorphan are easy to find, affordable for cash-strapped teens, and perfectly legal.

4. DXM abuse is common, according to recent studies, and easy access to OTC medications in stores and over the Internet probably contributes to this.

5. When consumed in large quantities, DXM can also cause hyperthermia, or high fever.

B1. Choose the appropriate words and fill in the blanks with their correct forms.

| lookout | strap | hyperthermia | slurred |
| impaired | stockpiling | antihistamine | narcotic |

1. _____ speech is an example of an anxiety symptom that can be incredibly frightening.

2. FDA clears addiction drug to treat patients addicted to _____ like heroin and morphine.

3. An _____ is a type of drug used to fight allergic reactions.

4. The poor was treated well in the hospital though he was _____ for cash.

5. The _____ may be fatal, and steps should be taken to dissipate heat quickly.

6. _____ dairy products is expensive and quality is difficult to maintain.

7. People should be on the _____ for symptoms of flu in winter.

8. 70% of people aged from 18 to 34 have experienced drumming in the ears, an obvious sign of _____ hearing.

B2. Match the following words with their English meaning

word	meaning
1. lookout	a. tie with string
2. strap	b. diminished in strength, quality, or utility
3. hyperthermia	c. spoken as if with a thick tongue
4. slurred	d. the act of looking out
5. impaired	e. accumulating and storing a reserve supply
6. stockpiling	f. abnormally high body temperature

B3. Fill in the blanks with the words in the text. The first letter is given to you

1. At a graduation party, it is common for students to encourage each other to c_____ a large mug of beer.

2. Hungry children often r_____ the cupboards for snacks while depressed teen-agers r_____ the medicine cabinet for cough suppressant to chug.

3. I've never i_____ hurt anyone.

4. Cigarettes can be an appetite s_____, and often smokers have a lower body weight than nonsmokers.

5. Certainly, there's plenty to worry about when it comes to how many calories we g_____ each day.

6. He v_____ all the food he had eaten.

7. Visually i_____ users cannot perceive this information, so there should be an alternative way for disabled users to be aware of the content.

C1. Choose the best answer for the following exercise

1. Please excuse me _____ your letter by mistake.

A. to open   B. to have opened   C. for opening   D. in opening

2. Certainly I posted your letter, and I remember _____ it.

A. posting   B. to post   C. to be posting   D. have posted

3. They must be at home, and there's a light _____ in the bedroom.

A. to shine   B. to be shining   C. shining   D. having shined

4. If the car won't start, _____ it.

A. try push   B. try pushing   C. to try pushing   D. to try to push

5. Mr. Smith dislikes _____ such clothes but his wife likes _____ them.

A. to wear, to wear   B. to wear, wearing

C. wearing, to wear   D. wearing, wear

6. _____ is a good form of exercise for both young and old.

A. Walk   B. Walking   C. The walk   D. To walk

7. When you're learning to drive, _____ a good teacher makes a big difference.

A. have   B. having   C. and have   D. and having

8. _____ this report _____ in such a short time was quite a difficult exercise.

A. Getting, done   B. Get, done

C. To get, to do   D. Getting, to do

9. I regret _____ what I said. I shouldn't have said it.

A. to say   B. saying   C. to be saying   D. said

10. I shall never forget _____ theAlps for the first time. It was really beautiful.

    A. to see   B. seeing   C. saw   D. being seeing

11. In the whole interview, he tried to avoid _____ their questions.

    A. to answer   B. answering

    C. to have answered   D. having answered

12. He was lucky and narrowly missed _____ .

    A. to injure   B. injuring   C. to be injured   D. being injured

13. I understand _____ to discuss the matter.

    A. your not wanting   B. not your wanting

    C. you not to want   D. you to not want

14. Don't be late. No one would like _____ .

    A. to be kept waiting   B. being keep waiting

    C. to be kept to wait   D. being kept to wait

15. He can't make himself _____ . His spoken English really needs

    _____ .

    A. understand, improving   B. understood, improving

    C. understand, to improve   D. understood, to improve

C2. Choose the best answer for the following exercises

1. The disc, digitally _____ in the studio, sounded fantastic at the party that night.

    A. recorded   B. recording   C. to be recorded   D. having recorded

2. Don't use words, expressions, or phrases _____ only to people with specific knowledge.

    A. being known   B. having been known

    C. to be known   D. known

3. A man is being questioned in relation to the _____ murder last night.

    A. advised   B. attended   C. attempted   D. admitted

4. The prize of the game show is $30,000 and an all expenses _____ vacation to China.

    A. paying   B. paid   C. to be paid   D. being paid

5. There have been several new events _____ to the program for the 2008 Beijing Olympic Games.

    A. add   B. to add   C. adding   D. added

6. Five people won the "China's Green Figure" award, a title _____ to ordinary people for their contributions to environmental protection.

    A. being given   B. is given   C. given   D. was given

7. "Things _____ never come again！" I couldn't help talking to myself.

　A. lost　　　　　B. losing　　　　　C. to lose　　　　　D. have lost

8. The first textbooks _____ for teaching English as a foreign language came out in the 16th century.

　A. having written　　　　　　　B. to be written

　C. being written　　　　　　　D. written

9. The trees _____ in the storm have been moved off the road.

　A. being blown down　　　　　　B. blown down

　C. blowing down　　　　　　　D. to blow down

10. The players _____ from the whole country are expected to bring us honor in this summer game.

　A. selecting　　B. to select　　　　C. selected　　　　D. having selected

11. We finished the run in less than half the time _____.

　A. allowing　　B. to allow　　　C. allowed　　　D. allows

12. It is one of the funniest things _____ on the Internet so far this year.

　A. finding　　B. being found　　C. to find　　　D. found

13. The repairs cost a lot，but it's money well _____.

　A. to spend　　B. spent　　　C. being spent　　D. spending

14. Now that we've discussed the steps _____ with this problem，are people happy?

　A. taking　　　B. take　　　　C. taken　　　　D. to take

15. I'm calling to enquire about the position _____ in yesterday's China Daily.

　A. advertised　　　　　　　　B. to be advertised

　C. advertising　　　　　　　　D. having advertised

16. The murderer was brought in，with his hands _____ behind his back.

　A. being tied　　B. having tied　　C. to be tied　　　D. tied

17. The managers discussed the plan that they would like to see _____ the next year.

　A. carry out　　　　　　　　B. carrying out

　C. carried out　　　　　　　　D. to carry out

18. Jenny hopes that Mr. Smith will suggest a good way to have her written English _____ in a short period.

　A. improved　　B. improving　　C. to improve　　D. improve

19. Even the best writers sometimes find themselves _____ for words.

　A. lose　　　B. at a loss　　　C. to lose　　　D. having lost

20. Michael put up a picture of Yao Ming beside the bed to keep himself _____

of his own dreams.

    A. reminding   B. to remind   C. reminded   D. remind

C3. Translate the following sentences into English.

1. 她有意不理我，继续做自己的工作。（intentionally）

2. 他病了很久，憔悴不堪。（seedy）

3. 她昨天胃不舒服，呕吐了几次。（vomit）

4. 尼古丁是香烟中的一种有毒物质。（nicotine）

5. 他那只受伤的胳膊不能抬起来。（impaired）

LISTENING

听力

Fill in the blanks according to what you hear.

What can you do for your cold or cough symptoms? Besides drinking plenty of fluids and getting plenty of rest, you may want to take medicines. There are lots of different cold and cough medicines, and they do different things.

1. Nasal decongestants – _____ .

2. Cough suppressants – _____ .

3. Expectorants – _____ .

4. Antihistamines – _____ .

5. Pain Relievers – _____ .

6. Here are some other things to keep in mind about cold and cough medicines. _____, because many cold and cough medicines contain the same active ingredients.

7. _____ can lead to serious injury. Do not give cough medicines to children under four, and don't give aspirin to children. Finally, antibiotics won't help a cold.

书网融合……

微课1   微课2   微课3   自测题

Unit 3 Peptic Disease

OBJECTIVES

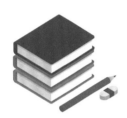

When you have completed Unit 3, you will be able to

⊙ understand and identify professional terms related to a peptic ulcer.

⊙ communicate with the doctor about some typical symptoms properly.

⊙ skim the passage for main idea.

⊙ describe the symptoms, the causes and the control of a peptic ulcer.

⊙ obtain information about a peptic ulcer by listening to the dialogue.

⊙ master the structure of attributive clause.

LEAD IN

When you experience abdominal discomfort, you may doubt you are having a peptic ulcer. Go through the following questions and if you get more than 5 "YES" answers to them, you need to be CAREFUL!

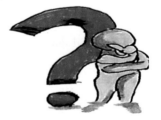

Q1: Do you have diffuse or localized abdominal pain?

Q2: Does the pain ever travel to the back or chest?

Q3: Do you have nausea associated with the pain?

Q4: Does eating make the pain better or worse?

Q5: Do you have black or bloody stools?

Q6: Do you ever vomit blood or material that looks like coffee grounds?

Q7: Do you take any medications (for example, pain relievers)?

Q8: Do you smoke cigarettes or drink alcohol?

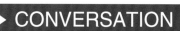 **CONVERSATION**

会话

Nicholas is a salesman and he has to have dinners with customers and drink a lot. Recently, he feels extremely uncomfortable in stomach. The following is a conversation he held with the doctor he visited.

Patient: Good morning, doctor.

Doctor: Good morning. Please sit down. What seems to be the matter?

Patient: I have a pain in the upper abdomen.

Doctor: What kind of pain is it?

Patient: It's kind of heartburn pain.

Doctor: How long have you had it?

Patient: I have had this kind of pain off and on for two years. Recently, it has got worse in frequency and severity.

Doctor: Do you often have alcohol?

Patient: Yes, I am a salesman. I have to have dinner with customers and drink a lot.

Doctor: Have you had any nausea or vomiting?

Patient: Yes, especially after I drink alcohol.

Doctor: What did you vomit, food or blood?

Patient: Food with a little blood.

Doctor: What was the color of the blood, red or black?

Patient: Like coffee.

Doctor: What's the color of your stool? Have you ever paid attention to it?

Patient: My stools have been black for the past two days and I feel weak.

Doctor: Have they ever been black before?

Patient: No. This is the first time.

Doctor: I'll examine your abdomen. Lie down on your back and loosen your clothes. Please bend your knees. (After a while) I think you've got a peptic ulcer. Most exactly, it might be a duodenal ulcer.

Patient: Then what should I do?

Doctor: I think we'd better take an X-ray film of your gastrointestinal tract. (writes a requisition form) When you leave here, go immediately to the Cashier's Office and give them this requisition. You will have to pay or show an insurance card. Then go to the department of radiology. You can wait for the results, then bring them back to me.

Patient: OK, thanks.

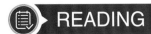 **READING**

Peptic Disease

Pre – reading

Is a peptic ulcer equivalent to erosion?

What are the causes of a peptic ulcer?

What are the symptoms of a peptic ulcer?

How do we diagnose the peptic ulcer?

While – reading

What Is a Peptic Ulcer? e 微课1

A peptic ulcer is a break in the inner lining of the esophagus, stomach, or duodenum. A peptic ulcer of the stomach is called a gastric ulcer; of the duodenum, a duodenal ulcer; and of the esophagus, an esophageal ulcer. Peptic ulcers occur when the lining of these organs is corroded by the acidic digestive (peptic) juices which are secreted by the cells of the stomach. A peptic ulcer differs from an erosion because it extends deeper into the lining of the esophagus, stomach, or duodenum and excites more of an inflammatory reaction from the tissues that are eroded.

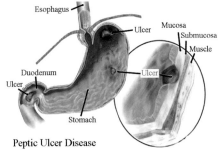

Peptic Ulcer Disease

Causes of Peptic Ulcers e 微课2

For many years, excess acid was believed to be the major cause of ulcer disease. Accordingly, the emphasis of treatment was on neutralizing and inhibiting the secretion of stomach acid. While acid is still considered necessary for the formation of ulcers, the two most important initiating causes of ulcers are infection of the stomach by a bacterium called "Helicobacter pyloricus" (H. pylori)[1] and chronic use of anti-inflammatory medications, commonly referred to as NSAIDs (nonsteroidal anti-inflammatory drugs)[2], including aspirin. Cigarette smoking also is an important cause of ulcer formation as well as failure of ulcer treatment.

Contrary to popular belief, alcohol, coffee, colas, spicy foods, and caffeine have no proven role in ulcer formation. Similarly, there is no conclusive evidence to suggest that life stresses or personality types contribute to ulcer disease.

Symptoms of Peptic Ulcers 🄴 微课3

Symptoms of ulcer disease are variable. Many ulcer patients experience minimal indigestion, abdominal discomfort that occurs after meals, or no discomfort at all. Some complain of upper abdominal burning or hunger pain one to three hours after meals or in the middle of the night. These symptoms often are promptly relieved by food or antacids that neutralize stomach acid. [3]The pain of ulcer disease correlates poorly with the presence or severity of active ulceration. Some patients have persistent pain even after an ulcer is almost completely healed by medication. Others experience no pain at all. Ulcers often come and go spontaneously without the individual ever knowing that they are present unless a serious complication (like bleeding or perforation) occurs.

Diagnosis of Peptic Ulcers

The diagnosis of an ulcer is made by either a barium upper gastrointestinal X-ray[4] (upper GI series) or an upper gastrointestinal endoscopy. [5]The barium upper GI X-ray is easy to perform and involves no risk or discomfort. However, barium X-rays are less accurate and may miss ulcers in up to 20% of the time.

An upper gastrointestinal endoscopy is more accurate than X-rays, but involves sedation of the patient and the insertion of a flexible tube through the mouth to inspect the esophagus, stomach, and duodenum. Upper endoscopy has the added advantage of having the capability of removing small tissue samples (biopsies) to test for H. pylori infection. Biopsies are also examined under a microscope to exclude a cancerous ulcer.

The Treatment for Peptic Ulcers

The goal of ulcer treatment is to relieve pain, heal the ulcer, and prevent complications. The first step in treatment involves the reduction of risk factors (NSAIDs and cigarettes). The next step is medications.

Summary

With modern treatment, patients with ulcer disease can lead normal lives without lifestyle changes or dietary restrictions. Cigarette smokers have been found to have more complications from ulcers and treatment failure. Eradication of the bacteria H. pylori not only heals ulcers but also prevents the recurrence of ulcer disease.

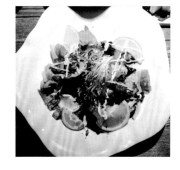

Notes

1. Helicobacterpyloricus（H. pylori）幽门螺杆菌。大量研究表明，超过90%的十二指肠溃疡和80%左右的胃溃疡，都是由幽门螺杆菌感染所导致的。

2. NSAIDs（non steroidal anti-inflammatory drugs）非甾体抗炎药，具有解热、镇痛和抗炎作用。本类药物起效迅速，可减轻炎症肿胀，解热，减轻疼痛并能改善功能，故临床应用广泛。

3. These symptoms often are promptly relieved by food or antacids that neutralize stomach acid.

这是一个含有限制性定语从句（attributive clause）的复杂句。主句是"These symptoms often are promptly relieved by food or antacids"，意思为"食物或解酸剂可以迅速减轻这些症状。""that neutralize stomach acid"作为一个限制性的定语从句来限定"food or antacid"，这样整个句子的意思就是"能够中和胃酸的食物或解酸剂可以迅速减轻这些症状。"

4. barium upper gastrointestinal X-ray：钡餐造影，是指用硫酸钡作为造影剂，在 X 线照射下显示消化道有无病变的一种检查方法。

5. upper gastrointestinal endoscopy：上消化道内窥镜检查，也叫做食管、胃、十二指肠镜检查或 EGD，是将一尖端带有灯光和摄像头的细小的管状物插入至上消化道进行观察，观察食管、胃和小肠的第一部分，十二指肠。

Glossary

Word	English definition	Example
corrode v.	cause to deteriorate due to the action of water, air, or an acid	Water corrodes metal
secrete v.	generate and separate from cells or bodily fluids	The kidneys secrete urine.
erosion n.	process of destroying or wearing away gradually	The erosion of the soil is damaging the forest
acidic adj.	being or containing an acid	Souse is believed to be highly acidic
neutralize v.	make ineffective by counterbalancing the effect of	This medicineneutralizes stomach acids
initiate v.	take the lead or initiative in	This term we will initiate a new teaching plan
variable adj.	something that is likely to vary or change	His mood is as variable as the weather
correlate v.	to have a close connection with something; to have a correlation to something	We can often correlate age with frequency of illness
persistent adj.	never-ceasing	His great success cannot depart from his persistent effort
spontaneous adj.	happening or arising without apparent external cause	It is a spontaneous cheer from the crowd

Word	English definition	Chinese definition
peptic ulcer n.	an ulcer of the mucous membrane lining of the alimentary tract	消化性溃疡
esophagus n.	the passage between the pharynx and the stomach	食道

Word	English definition	Chinese definition
duodenum *n.*	the part of the small intestine between the stomach and the jejunum	十二指肠
gastric *adj.*	relating to or involving the stomach	胃的
inflammatory *adj.*	of inflammation，that is，a response of body tissues to injury or irritation；characterized by pain and swelling and redness and heat	发炎的
indigestion *n.*	a disorder of digestive function characterized by discomfort or heartburn or nausea	消化不良
antacids *n.*	an agent that counteracts or neutralizes acidity（especially in the stomach）	解酸剂
complication *n.*	any disease or disorder that occurs during the course of（or because of）another disease	并发症
perforation *n.*	a hole made in something	穿孔
gastrointestinal *adj.*	of or relating to the stomach and intestines	胃肠的
endoscopy *n.*	visual examination of the interior of a hollow body organ by use of an endoscope	内诊镜检查
sedation *n.*	the administration of a sedative agent or drug	镇静
biopsies *n.*	examination of tissues or liquids from the living body to determine the existence or cause of a disease	活组织检查

Post – reading

A1. Complete the following "Peptic Ulcer Disease at A Glance" with proper words.

Peptic ulcers can affect the stomach，1 _____，or esophagus. Peptic ulcer formation is related to 2 _____ bacteria in the stomach，anti-inflammatory medications，and smoking cigarettes. Ulcer pain may not correlate with the presence or severity of 3 _____ . Diagnosis of ulcer is made with 4 _____ or endoscopy. Complications of ulcers include 5 _____，perforation，and blockage of the stomach. Treatment of ulcers involves 6 _____ combinations to eradicate H. pylori，eliminating risk factors，stomach acid suppression with medications，and preventing complications.

A2. Answer following questions.

1. What is a peptic ulcer?

2. What are the three major causes of peptic ulcers?

3. Is the pain of ulcer disease closely related to the presence or severity of activeulceration?

4. A patient wants to have an accurate diagnosis of an ulcer，which is between the barium upper gastrointestinal X-ray and upper gastrointestinal endoscopy. What is the preferable meth-

od of diagnosis?

5. Are cigarettes a risk factor in peptic diseases?

B1. Fill in the blanks with the words from the box. Change the form if necessary.

eradicate	corrode	correlate	interfere
develop	spontaneous	counteract	digest

1. What the society must immediately address is to minimize the quantity of any fake commodities and ＿＿＿＿＿＿ any opportunities to manufacture them.

2. It was designed to be a material with high ＿＿＿＿＿＿ resistance and strength over a wide temperature range.

3. These are the times of fast foods and slow ＿＿＿＿＿＿; tall men, and short character; steep profits and shallow relationships.

4. Indoor activities are somewhat challenging as well. There are chess and book reading which can also ＿＿＿＿＿＿ our minds.

5. The ＿＿＿＿＿＿ outpouring of generosity from individual Chinese in the last two weeks should be a source of pride to us all.

6. Don't expend your right limitlessly; don't ＿＿＿＿＿＿ others' ideals and beliefs; don't think yourself more foresighted than others.

7. The Chinese government has raised the urban minimum living allowance for low-income-families by 15 Yuan a month to try and ＿＿＿＿＿＿ the recent inflation of daily commodities.

8. A growing body of research has found that changes in sunspot activity directly ＿＿＿＿＿＿ with temperature changes on Earth.

B2. Match the words with their synonyms.

1. corrode	a) start, begin
2. secrete	b) continue, keep at
3. neutralize	c) changeable
4. variable	d) produce
5. initiate	e) deteriorate, rot
6. correlate	f) automatic
7. persist	g) counteract
8. spontaneous	h) associate, link

B3. Fill in the blanks with the words in the text. The first letter is given to you.

1. We i＿＿＿＿＿＿ reforms and opening more than 20 years ago.

2. His mood is as v＿＿＿＿＿＿ as the weather.

3. Honey should not be stored in a metallic container because of it's a＿＿＿＿＿＿ na-

ture，and corrodes the metal easily.

4. Weisen-U can n_____ stomachic acid to treat peptic ulcer.

5. Tree-planting helps to conserve water and prevent soil e_____ .

6. If insomnia is p_____ , visit your doctor.

7. Tears are s_____ by an organ under the upper eyelid.

C1. Study the following medical affix，decide its meaning，and match more words that end with the same affix with their Chinese equivalents.

C1 – 1 endoscopy

The word "endoscopy" contains an affix "endo". What does it mean?

1. endoscopy	a）内分泌
2. endocrine	b）内窥镜
3. endocardium	c）向心的
4. endocentric	d）心内膜

C1 – 2 pylori

The above word "pylori" is the plural form of the word "pylorus" .

1. pylorus	a）Pylori 幽门
2. fungus	b）Abaci 算盘
3. abacus	c）Cacti 仙人掌
4. cactus	d）Fungi 真菌

C2. Fill in the blanks with appropriate relative pronouns and point out the attributive clauses in the passage.

This Charming Property

People 1 _____ tell the truth about the properties they are selling should be given prizes for honesty. A house 2 _____ is described as "spacious" will be found to be too large. Words like "enchanting" "delightful" "convenient" "attractive"，3 _____ are commonly used all mean "small" . The words "small" and "picturesque"，4 _____ are not so frequently used，both mean "too small" . A "picturesque house" is one with a bedroom 5 _____ is too small to put a bed in and a kitchen 6 _____ is too small to boil an egg in. My prize for honesty goes to someone 7 _____ recently described a house he was selling in the following way："This house，8 _____ is situated in a very rough area of London，is really in need of repair. The house，9 _____ has a terrible lounge and a tiny dining room also has three miserable bedrooms and a bathroom 10 _____ is fitted with a leaky shower. The central heating，11 _____ is expensive to run，is unreliable. The neighbors，12 _____ are generally unfriendly, are not likely to welcome you. This property, 13 _____ is definitely not recommended, is ridiculously overpriced at £ 85, 000. ”

C3. Translate the following sentences into English.

1. 这种酸能腐蚀铁。（corrode）

2. 健康与膳食平衡有关。（correlate）

3. 火山爆发是自然产生的。（spontaneous）

4. 持续的咳嗽可能是肺炎的症状。（persistent）

5. 肺炎是我们最害怕的并发症。（complication）

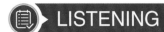 LISTENING

听力

Complete the sentences with the words you hear.

Patient: Doctor, here is the result.

Doctor: OK. Let me see. The X-ray doctor found 1 _____ and distortion of the duodenum although there was no actual visible 2 _____ on the X-ray. This does not necessarily mean that you have no ulcer. Let me give you a gastroscopy.

Patient: I heard that it was really 3 _____ to have a gastroscopy. How is it done?

Doctor: Don't worry. It will be over soon. I will pass a hollow tube equipped with a 4 _____ called endoscope down your 5 _____ and into your esophagus, stomach and small intestine. Using the 6 _____, I try to look for ulcers.

Patient: Oh, gosh! It's terrible.

Doctor: This is good for your 7 _____. Don't be afraid. Did you have your 8 _____ this morning?

Patient: No.

Doctor: How about after 8 o'clock last night?

Patient: No, I had nothing after supper at 6 o'clock, even 9 _____.

Doctor: That's fine. Do you need to do it under a local 10 _____.

Patient: That will make me feel less painful?

Doctor: Yes, just like sleeping. After sleeping, it will be over.

Patient: OK.

书网融合······

微课1　　　　微课2　　　　微课3　　　　自测题

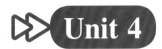 **Unit 4** **Constipation**

PPT

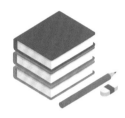

OBJECTIVES

When you have completed Unit 4, you will be able to

⊙ understand and identify professional terms related to constipation.

⊙ communicate with the doctor about some typical symptoms properly.

⊙ skim the passage for main idea.

⊙ describe the symptoms, the causes and the control ofconstipation.

⊙ obtain information about constipation by listening to the dialogue.

⊙ master the structure of adverbial clauses of condition.

LEAD IN

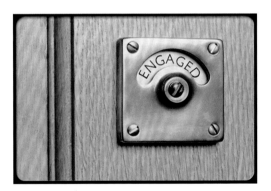

What does "engaged" mean if it is a toilet booth?

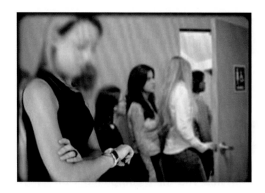

What are the possible reasons for such a long queue in a toilet?

CONVERSATION

会话

Sandra is a mom of a 2 - year old boy. She's been worried these days because her boy, Alex, seems suffering from having constipation. She's visiting Alex's pediatrician Neil for help. What are some ways of easing constipation in children?

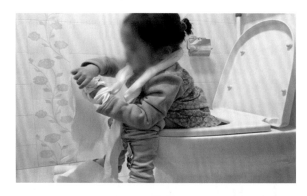

Sandra: Good morning, Doctor. It seems like Alex is constipated. I'm really worried.

Neil: Take it easy. We do not call it constipation until he is having bowel movements less than 3 times per week. So Alex, Could you tell me how long has it been since you passed stools?

Alex (a little confused by the question and looks at his mom): Mom?

Sandra: Oh, it's been three days.

Neil: Does he have any abdominal pain or cramps?

Sandra: No. He feels no pain in any part of his stomach, and he has good appetite.

Neil: Does he drink a lot of water every day?

Sandra: No. He is reluctant to drink water.

Neil: You must ask Alex to drink enough water. It helps to pass the stool. Does he hold back bowel movements?

Sandra: Yes. It seems he is not ready for toilet training. What should I do?

Neil：You can buy a potty for him. Tell him that belongs to him. He can decorate it with his favorite stickers. Praise him once he sits on it when he feels the urge of passing stools. Gradually, he will be used to the potty and he will be proud of being able to pass stools himself.

Sandra：Thank you, doctor. What else can I do to ease his constipation?

Neil：It's ordinary for children to not pass stools for two days. Don't call it constipation or otherwise you'll stress him too much.

Sandra：I see. We should relax a little bit about this issue.

Neil：That's right. Another thing we can do is to get enough fiber in his diet. Vegetables, fresh fruits, dried fruits, and whole wheat, or oatmeal cereals are excellent sources of fiber. With enough water, enough dietary fiber, and regular physical activities, Alex will be fine soon.

Sandra：Thank you so much, doctor. Bye-bye.

Neil：Bye-bye.

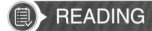 **READING**

Constipation

Pre – reading

Is there a definite definition of constipation?

Medically speaking, what is a severe constipation?

How to distinguish acute constipation from a chronic one?

While – reading

> ### What Is Constipation?
>
> Constipation means different things to different people. For many people, it simply means infrequent stools. For others, however, constipation means hard stools, difficulty passing stools (straining), or a sense of incomplete emptying after a bowel movement. The cause of each of these "types" of constipation probably is different, and the approach to each should be tailored to the specific type of constipation. [1] Constipation also can alternate with diarrhea.
>
> This pattern commonly occurs as part of Irritable Bowel Syndrome (IBS). At the extreme end of the constipation spectrum is fecal impaction, a condition in which stool hardens in the rectum and prevents the passage of any stool.

The Number of Bowel Movements

The number of bowel movements generally decreases with age. Ninety-five percent of adults have bowel movements between three and 21 times per week, and this would be considered normal. The most regular pattern is one bowel movement a day, but this pattern is seen in less than 50% of people. Moreover, most people are irregular and do not have bowel movements every day or the same number of bowel movements each day.

Medical Definition of Constipation

Medically speaking, constipation usually is defined as fewer than three bowel movements per week. Severe constipation is defined as less than one bowel movement per week. There is no medical reason to have a bowel movement every day. Going without a bowel movement for two or three days does not cause physical discomfort, only mental distress for some people. Contrary to popular belief, there is no evidence that "toxins" accumulate when bowel movements are infrequent or that constipation leads to cancer.

Acute or Chronic?

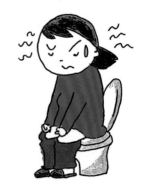

It is important to distinguish acute constipation from chronic constipation. Acute constipation requires urgent assessment because a serious medical illness may be the underlying cause (for example, tumors of the colon). Constipation also requires an immediate assessment if it is accompanied by worrisome symptoms such as rectal bleeding, abdominal pain and cramps, nausea and vomiting, as well as involuntary loss of weight. [2]

In contrast, the evaluation of chronic constipation may not be urgent, particularly if simple measures bring relief.

Means of Medical Evaluation

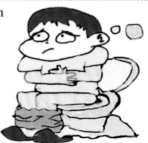

Medical evaluation of constipation may include a history, physical examination, blood tests, abdominal X-rays, barium enema, colonic transit studies, [3] defecography, [4] anorectal motility studies, [5] and colonic motility studies.

> ### Treatment of Constipation
>
> Treatment of constipation may include dietary fiber, non-stimulant laxatives, stimulant laxatives, enemas, suppositories, biofeedback training,[6] and surgery.
>
> Stimulant laxatives should be used as a last resort because of the possibility that they may permanently damage the colon and worsen constipation. Most herbal laxatives contain stimulant-type laxatives and should be used, if at all, as a last resort.

Notes

1. The cause of each of these "types" of constipation probably is different, and the approach to each should be tailored to the specific type of constipation.

此句中的 be tailored to 是 tailor sth to/for sb/sth 的被动形式，表示"专门制作；订做"的意思。整句话表示"每一种类型的便秘成因可能是不一样的，所以具体到每一种便秘的解决方法也应该因情况而定。"

2. Constipation also requires an immediate assessment if it is accompanied by worrisome symptoms such as rectal bleeding, abdominal pain and cramps, nausea and vomiting, and involuntary loss of weight.

该句是一个含有条件状语从句的复杂句。主句是"Acute constipation also requires an immediate assessment"。在理解复杂句时，我们要先把握主句的意思。

3. colonic transit studies 结肠传输试验

4. defecography 排粪造影

5. anorectal motility studies 肛门直肠能动性试验

6. biofeedback training 生物反馈训练

Glossary

Word	English definition	Example
infrequent *adj.*	not often, not occurring regularly or at short intervals	Pregnancies in women over the age of 45 are infrequent
tailor *v.*	adjust to a specific need or a market	We can tailor our design to meet your request
alternate *v.*	go back and forth, swing back and forth between two states or conditions	Sunny weather alternated with rain
irritable *adj.*	easily annoyed	Our teacher is an irritable old lady. She gets angry easily
spectrum *n.*	full or wide range or sequence	There is a wide spectrum of opinions on this problem
accumulate *v.*	collect or gather	Dust and dirt soon accumulate if a house is not cleaned regularly
distinguish *v.*	detect with the senses	An experienced physician can distinguish illness from health by a visual examination of the tongue

续表

Word	English definition	Chinese definition
acute *adj.*	having a rapid onset and short but severe course	急性的
chronic *adj.*	being long lasting and recurrent	慢性的
stimulant *n.*	a drug that temporarily quickens some vital process	兴奋剂
stool *n.*	solid excretory product evacuated from bowels	粪便
bowel *n.*	the part of the alimentary canal between the stomach and the anus	肠
diarrhea *n.*	frequent and watery bowel movement	腹泻
fecal impaction *n.*	accumulation of hardened faces in the rectum or lower colon which the person cannot move	粪便嵌塞
rectum *n.*	the terminal section of alimentary canal	直肠
toxins *n.*	a poisonous substance produced during the metabolic process	毒素
tumor *n.*	an abnormal new mass of tissues that serves no purpose	肿瘤、肿块
colon *n.*	the part of the large intestine between the cecum and the rectum	结肠
abdominal *adj.*	of or relating to or near the abdomen	腹部的
barium enema	injection of a liquid through the anus to stimulate evacuation; sometimes used for diagnostic purposes	钡灌肠
laxative *n.*	food or medicine that you take to make you go to the toilet	泻药
suppository *n.*	a small plug of medication designed for insertion into the rectum or vagina where it melts	栓剂

Post – reading

A1. Yes/No/Not Given Questions.

Refer to the passage and look at the statements below. Write

YES   if the statement agrees with the writer;

NO   if the statement does not agree with the writer;

NOT GIVEN   if there is no information about this in the passage.

1. Constipation means infrequent stools.

2. If one patient is suffering from constipation and diarrhea alternatively, he/she is having IBS.

3. 50% of people do not have bowel movements every day.

4. Toxins will accumulate when bowel movements are infrequent.

5. Acute constipation requires urgent assessment.

6. Abdominal pain and cramps do not go with constipation.

7. Use of stimulant laxatives is not encouraged.

8. However, herbal laxatives can be used since they are herbal and contain no stimulant.

A2. Answer the following questions.

1. What does constipation mean?

2. What does IBS stand for?

3. What's the relationship between the number of bowel movements and age?

4. What is the medical definition of constipation?

5. Is the use of laxatives encouraged by doctor?

B1. Choose the appropriate words and fill in the blanks with their correct forms.

alternate	tailor	acute	frequent
irritate	accumulate	chronic	stimulant

1. Her mood _____ between happiness and despair.

2. Coffee and tea are mild _____ .

3. _____ appendicitis requires immediate surgery.

4. Her calls became less _____ .

5. Some painkilling drugs can _____ the lining of the stomach.

6. Special programs of study are _____ to the needs of specific groups.

7. I seem to have _____ a lot of books through years of reading.

8. The air quality is so poor that it's terrible for patients of _____ bronchitis.

B2. Find appropriate words from the text to describe the following pictures.

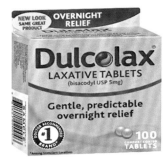
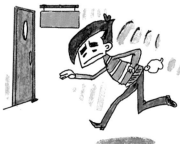
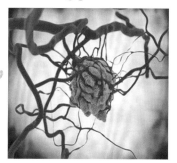

_____   _____   _____

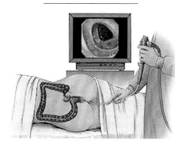
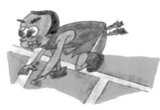
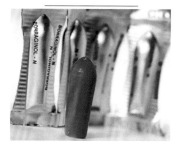

_____   _____   _____

B3. Fill in the blanks with the words in the text. The first letter is given to you.

1. The doctor said that his father had a _____ appendicitis and should be operated immediately.

2. Dust and dirt soon a _____ if a house is not cleaned regularly.

3. The twins are so much alike that it is impossible to d _____ one from another.

4. We were both workaholics who got more i _____ when we were exhausted.

5. Rememberthat most babies with i _____ BMs are not truly " constipated " and nothing needs to be changed.

6. Her aggressive moods a _____ with gentle or more co-operative states.

C1. Study the following medical affix, decide its meaning, and then match more words that end with the same affix to their Chinese equivalents.

C1 – 1 defecography

The word "defecography" contains an affix "graphy". What does it mean?

1. angiography	a）心电图
2. photography	b）血管造影
3. electrocardiography	c）亲笔签名
4. autography	d）照相

C1 – 2 barium

The above word "barium" contains "ium". What does it mean?

1. sodium	a）镁
2. potassium	b）钙
3. calcium	c）钾
4. magnesium	d）钠

C2. Fill in the blanks with appropriate forms of the given verbs and pay attention to the adverbial clauses of condition.

The Secret of a Long Life

Grygori Pilikian recently celebrated his 114th birthday, and reporters visited him in his mountain village in Georgia to find out the secret of a long life. "The secret of a long life," Grygori said, "is happiness. If you (be) _____ happy, you will live a long time. " "Are you married?" a reporter asked. "Yes," Grygori replied. "I married my third wife when I was 102. If you are happily married, you (live) _____ forever. But for my third wife, I (die) _____ years ago. " "What about smoking and drinking?" a reporter asked. "Yes, they are important," Grygori said. "Don't smoke at all and you (feel) _____ well. Drink two glasses of wine a day and you (be) _____ healthy and happy. "   " If you (can/live) _____ you life again, what (you/do) _____ ?" a reporter asked. "I would do what I have done. If I had had more sense, I (eat) _____ more yoghourt!" he chuckled. "Supposing you (can/change) _____ one thing in your life what (you/change) _____ ?" another reporter asked. "Not much," Grygori replied. "So you don't have any regrets?" "Yes, I have one regret," Grygori replied. "If I (know) ＿＿＿＿＿＿ I was going to live so long, I (look after) ＿＿＿＿＿＿ myself better!"

C3. Translate the following sentences into English.

1. 王老师上周上了二十节课，太累了以至于患上了急性咽喉炎。(acute)

2. 工作和休息应交替进行。(alternate)

3. 长期的艰苦工作使他患上了慢性胃炎。(chronic)

4. 尽管茶和咖啡是温和的兴奋剂，睡觉前最好也不要喝。(stimulant)

5. 我昨天晚上失眠了，所以今天的脾气很急躁。(irritable)

LISTENING

听力

Complete the sentences with the words you hear.

1. Our bodies are ＿＿＿＿＿＿ to trillions of other organisms that influence our health and probably our ＿＿＿＿＿＿ .

2. Researchers found that mice given gut microbes (肠道微生物) from ＿＿＿＿＿＿ humans became fatter than those that got microbes carried by ＿＿＿＿＿＿ folks.

3. When the husky and lean mice shared microbes (微生物) with each other, the bigger ones picked up some of the beneficial gut flora and had improved ＿＿＿＿＿＿ .

4. But this shift only occurred if the mice were on a high-fiber, low-saturated fat (低饱和脂肪) ＿＿＿＿＿＿ .

5. It's not clear how humans might ＿＿＿＿＿＿ our microbial communities (微生物群) to change health or ＿＿＿＿＿＿ class.

6. The mice in the study were raised in ＿＿＿＿＿＿ environments and had no native microbiomes (原生微生物) of their own. In people, so-called fecal transplants have been reserved for more severe conditions than a bulging belly. And probiotic products (益生菌产品), such as yogurt, are minimally effective.

7. But ＿＿＿＿＿＿ or ＿＿＿＿＿＿ , what your belly looks like on the outside might have a lot to do with what's on the inside.

书网融合……

 微课1　　　微课2　　　微课3　　　自测题

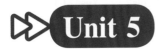

Unit 5 — Urinary Tract Infection

PPT

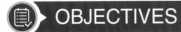

OBJECTIVES

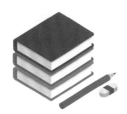

When you have completed Unit 5, you will be able to

⊙ understand and identify professional terms related to UTI.

⊙ communicate with the doctor about some typical symptoms properly.

⊙ skim the passage for main idea.

⊙ describe the symptoms, the causes and the control of UTI.

⊙ obtain information about UTI by listening to the lecture.

⊙ master the structure "*no matter* + *who*, *what*, *where*, *when*, *how*, *if*, *whether*".

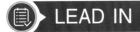

LEAD IN

Answer the question

Q: What do you do five to six times a day but never think twice about?

A: ⋯⋯

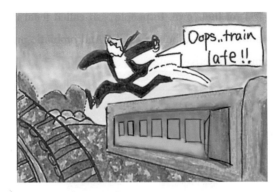

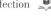

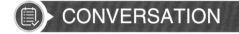 **CONVERSATION**

会话

Ted feels pain when he goes to the bathroom，so he goes to the drug's store directly.

Pharmacist：May I help you？

Ted：I'm running a temperature，and I feel pain when urinating.

Pharmacist：Where do you feel pain？

Ted：In the abdomen.

Pharmacist：Did you urinate more often than usual？

Ted：Yes.

Pharmacist：What color is your urine？

Ted：Cloudy.

Pharmacist：Have you been ill like this before？

Ted：Yes. I had a Urinary Tract Infection last year. I'm so busy right now，and I know I don't have enough rest or drink enough water. I think I'm making myself ill again.

Pharmacist：I think you are right.

Ted：The drugs which were previously bought from the hospital are out of date，so I come here directly to buy some.

Pharmacist：I'm sorry. I cannot sell you any antibiotic without a doctor's certificate or prescription.

Ted：Really？But I've had this illness before. I know what I have to do. There is no need for me to go and see a doctor again. That's a waste of time. I've a lot of work to do.

Pharmacist：Nothing is more important than your health！Right？This is a regulation which is made by the State Food and Drug Administration. We must comply with it.

Ted：I understand.

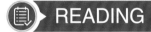 **READING**

Urinary Tract Infections

Pre – reading

How many times do you go to the bathroom each day？

What causes frequent urination？

How is it treated？

While – reading

What Exactly Is a Urinary Tract?

Your urinary tract is actually a system made up of these main parts：

1. two kidneys 2. two ureters 3. bladder 4. urethra

All day long, the kidneys clean waste products from your blood. The waste becomes urine (pee), which drips into the ureters (long, thin tubes, one connected to each kidney). From there, the urine travels through the ureters down to the bladder.

When it's empty, your bladder is about the same size as an empty balloon[1]. It looks like one, too! Then the bladder slowly fills up with the urine coming from the kidneys. When you have about a cup (237 milliliters) of urine in your bladder, your brain tells you it's time to find a bathroom.

Once you're ready to pee, you relax a set of muscles at the bottom of your bladder. That lets the urine rush into the urethra, a tube that leads from your bladder out of your body.

Ah！That feels better.

Urinary Tract Troubles

Girls are more likely than boys to get a Urinary Tract Infection (UTI). That's because their urethras are much shorter than boys' urethras. The shorter urethra means bacteria can get up into the bladder more easily and cause an infection there. Some of the bacteria that cause UTIs normally live in your intestines. Each time you have a bowel movement (poop), some of these bacteria come out of your body. If the bacteria aren't wiped away properly, they stay on your skin. In girls, this means they can grow near the opening of the urethra because their urethras are closer to where they wipe. [2] From there, bacteria can get inside the urethra, causing irritation. [3] This is called Urethritis. It's just a hop, skip, and a jump from the urethra to the bladder. If the bacteria go there, they can cause a bladder infection, which is a type of UTI. You may also hear a bladder infection called Cystitis, which really means an irritation of the bladder. Sometimes the harmful bacteria keep spreading. From the bladder, they may head into one of the ureters and climb up into a kidney. This type of UTI is called Pyelonephritis, or a kidney infection, and it's serious because it can damage the kidneys and make you very sick.

How Do I Know if I Have a UTI?

You may notice signs of a Urinary Tract Infection before anyone else can see there's anything wrong with you. That's why it's important to talk with the parent if you're having peeing problems. Ask yourself these questions and share your answers with your mom or dad：

⊙ Does it hurt or sting when you pee?

⊙ Can you only pee a little bit at a time?

⊙ Do you have to get up many times in the night to pee?

⊙ Is your pee cloudy?

⊙ Does it smell bad when you pee?

These are signs and symptoms of a bladder infection，so based on your answers，your mom or dad may decide to call your doctor or take you in for a visit.

Also be sure to tell a parent if you have of those symptoms，plus you feel the chills，or have pain in your belly or back，just have under your lower ribs. These are signs of a kidney infection and you should see a doctor right away.

Bye-Bye，UTI

Once you've had a UTI, you'll never want to have one again！To help keeping those bacteria out of your urinary tract，take these steps：

⊙ Keep clean.

⊙ Don't hold it. If you have to go.

⊙ When you're thirsty，drink something，no matter how busy you are. [4] Water and cranberry extract are two good choices.

⊙ Wear cotton underwear.

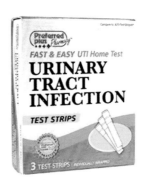

Nylon underwear traps moisture near your body，especially when it's hot outside. Bacteria love to grow in warm，moist feverish places.

Notes

1. When it's empty，your bladder is about the same size as an empty balloon.

"the same size as"意思为"与…一样大"，即以前学过的"as…as…"结构。如：这件大衣与那件大衣一样长。This coat is as long as that one. = This coat is the same size as that one.

2. In girls，this means they［bacteria］can grow near the opening of the urethra because their urethras are closer to where they wipe.

此句中注意 to 后的 where they wipe 为介词后的宾语从句，非地点状语从句。宾语从句之所以称其为宾语从句是因为整个从句在大句子中做宾语。总体而言有三种情况，可以带宾语。1）及物动词后跟从句，即为宾语从句。如：I don't know where he is from. 2）介词后跟从句，即为宾语从句。如：She walked over to where he sat. 3）be + adj. 后跟从句，可为宾语从句。如：I am not sure what I ought to do.

3. From there, bacteria can get inside the urethra, causing irritation (to the urethra).

"causing…" 为现在分词作结果状语。动词的 – ing 形式作状语，可以表示时间、原因、结果、条件、让步、行为方式、伴随状况等。如：He comes home late every evening, making his wife very angry.

= He comes home late every evening, which makes his wife very angry.

= He comes home late every evening, and it makes his wife very angry.

4. When you are thirsty, drink something, no matter how busy you are. 微课 1

"no matter + 疑问词 who, what, where, when, how, if, whether" 意为"无论，不管"。如：No matter where you work, you can always find time to study. 该结构需注意三点：①时态：主将从现的方式表将来。如：No matter when he comes again, he'll be welcome. ②被修饰的名词或形容词、副词需紧跟在 no matter 之后，置于主语之前。如：We'll have to find the job, no matter how long it takes. ③no matter who, what, when 引导让步状语从句时，可与 whoever, whatever, whenever 换用。如：

No matter who knocks, don't open the door.

= Whoever knocks, don't open the door.

Glossary

Word	English definition	Example
pee n. /v.	When someone pees, they urinate	He needed to pee
poop n. /v.	to get rid offaeces from your body	Whales poop at the surface
sting n. /v.	a kind of pain; cause a sharp or stinging pain or discomfort	Some medicated sprays can sting sensitive skin
feverish adj.	of or relating to or characterized by fever	A feverish child refuses to eat and asks only for cold drinks
chill n.	coldness due to a cold environment	September is here, bringing with it a chill in the mornings
rib n.	any of the 12 pairs of curved arches of bone extending from the spine to or toward the sternum in humans (and similar bones in most vertebrates)	The goalkeeper was taken off in a stretcher with a rib injury just before half-time
cranberry n.	red berries with a sour taste	Wisconsin is expected to be the top cranberry producer this year
extract v. /n.	a solution obtained by steeping or soaking a substance (usually in water)	Blend in the lemon extract, lemon peel and walnuts
trap n. /v.	to hold something inside so it cannot escape, as in a trap	Holes in teeth trap food particles and decay sets in causing dental cavities
moisture n.	wetness caused by water	When the soil is dry, more moisture is lost from the plant

续表

Word	English definition	Chinese definition
urine *n.*	the liquid that you get rid of from your body when you go to the toilet	尿
bacteria *n.*	very small organisms. Some can cause disease.	细菌
urinary tract *n.*	the organs and tubes involved in the production and excretion of urine	尿路
ureter *n.*	either of a pair of thick-walled tubes that carry urine from the kidney to the urinary bladder	尿管
symptom *n.*	any sensation or change in bodily function that is experienced by a patient and is associated with a particular disease	症状
bladder *n.*	a soft bag that is filled with water or air like the organ in the body that holds urine after it passes through the kidneys and before it leaves the body	膀胱
urethra *n.*	duct through which urine is discharged in most mammals and which serves as the male genital duct	尿道
infection *n.*	a disease caused by germs that enter the body	传染，感染 微课2
intestine *n.*	the part of the alimentary canal between the stomach and the anus	肠
bowel *n.*	the long tube in the body that helps digest food and carries solid waste out of the body	肠
irritation	(pathology) abnormal sensitivity to stimulation	刺激性
urethritis *n.*	inflammation of the urethra; results in painful urination	尿道炎 微课3
cystitis *n.*	inflammation of the urinary bladder and ureters	膀胱炎
pyelonephritis *n.*	inflammation of the kidney and its pelvis caused by bacterial infection	肾盂肾炎

Post – reading

A1. Answer the questions briefly.

1. How many main parts does your urinary tract include? List these parts.

2. When can your brain know it's time to find a bathroom?

3. Who are more prone (more likely) to get a UTI?

4. What are the signs and symptoms of a bladder infection?

A2. Scan and complete the sentences.

1. UTIs can be divided into _____, _____, and _____.

2. In the first, _____ aren't wiped away properly, so they stay on the skin and get inside _____, causing _____ to it.

3. When the bacteria jump from _____ to _____, it means an

_____ to the bladder.

4. If _____ climb up into _____, it becomes pyelonephritis which is much more serious.

B1. Choose the appropriate words and fill in the blanks with their correct forms.

sting	irritation	feverish
chill	extract	trap

1. Citric acid can be _____ from the juice of oranges, lemons, limes or grapefruit.

2. Her skin felt moist and _____.

3. This won't hurt — you will just feel a little _____.

4. This is an _____ and inflammation of the edge of the eyelid.

5. I would hate him to think I'm trying to _____ him.

6. The violence used against the students sent a _____ through Indonesia.

B2. Write down the words with the help of pictures.

1. _____ 2. _____ 3. _____ 4. _____

B3. Guess the meaning from prefix and suffix.

– itis = inflammation 炎症

myocarditis 心肌炎   bronchitis 支气管炎   tonsillitis   扁桃体炎

meningitis _____   rachitis _____   rhinitis _____

C1. Multiple choice

1. After _____ seemed like half an hour, the teacher gave us the correct answer.

   A. that   B. what   C. which   D. it

2. I know nothing about the accident except _____ I read in the newspaper.

   A. that   B. which   C. what   D. whether

3. People were more honest a long time ago, when life was very different from

_____ it is today.

　A. which　　　　B. that　　　　　C. what　　　　　D. how

4. She was never satisfied with _____ she had achieved.

　A. that　　　　　B. which　　　　　C. what　　　　　D. whether

5. No one had told Smith about _____ a lecture the following day.

　A. there being　　　　　　　　　B. there be

　C. there would be　　　　　　　　D. there was

6. Before I went downstairs, I had prepared myself very carefully _____ .

　A. with which　　B. for what　　　C. with what　　　D. for that

7. We can assign the work to _____ is reliable.

　A. who　　　　　B. whoever　　　　C. whom　　　　　D. whomever

C2. Multiple choice

1. _____ from heart trouble for years, Professor White has to take some medicine with him wherever he goes.

　A. Suffered　　　　　　　　　　B. Suffering

　C. Having suffered　　　　　　　D. Being suffered

2. Finding her car stolen, _____ .

　A. a policeman was asked to help

　B. the area was searched thoroughly

　C. it was looked for everywhere

　D. she hurried to a policeman for help

3. He sent me an e-mail, _____ to get further information.

　A. hoped　　　　B. hoping　　　　C. to hope　　　　D. hope

4. While building a tunnel through the mountain, _____ .

　A. an underground lake was discovered

　B. there was an underground lake discovered

　C. a lake was discovered underground

　D. the workers discovered an underground lake

5. Suddenly, a tall man driving a golden carriage _____ the girl and took her away, _____ into the woods.

　A. seizing; disappeared　　　　　B. seized; disappeared

　C. seizing; disappearing　　　　　D. seized; disappearing

C3. Rewrite the sentences using the " – ing" form

1. His father died. His father left him a lot of money.

_____

2. She was so angry that she threw the toy on the ground.

She broke it into pieces.

___

C4. Multiple choice

1. _____ team wins on Saturday will go through to the national championships.

    A. No matter what   B. No matter which

    C. Whatever   D. Whichever

2. _____ we gave him something to eat，he would save it up for his little sister.

    A. Whatever   B. However   C. Whenever   D. Whichever

3. Doctor Godwin saysthat _____ what forceful arguments against cigarettes there are，many people insist on smoking.

    A. though   B. however   C. no matter   D. even if

4. _____ , Mother will wait for him to have dinner.

    A. However late is he   B. However he is late

    C. However is he late   D. However late he is

5. ——Could you do me a favor?

    ——It depends on _____ it is.

    A. which   B. whichever   C. what   D. whatever

6. The old tower must be saved，_____ the cost.

    A. however   B. whatever   C. whichever   D. wherever

C5. Translation

1. 不管我干得多么卖力，总是有做不完的工作。(no matter…)

2. 他把杯子掉了，结果摔得粉碎。(- ing)

3. Linda 的钱包款式与 Jimmy 的一模一样。(the same… as…)

4. 我不知该从何开始。(where…)

5. 细菌喜欢在温暖潮湿的地方生长。(love …)

📋 ▶ LISTENING

听力

Part A   You are going to hear a report on UTIs. Refer to the listening and look at the statements below. Write

True   if the statement agrees with the listening material；

False   if the statement does not agree with the listening material.

1. About 5 million people per year are affected by UTIs.

2. Men are more likely to get UTIs than women.

3. The urinary tract's exposure to contaminants provides greater opportunities for organisms to grow and survive.

4. Antibiotic therapy can be initiated after the diagnosis has been confirmed.

5. Increasing fluid intake has no effect on UTIs.

Part B　Complete the sentences.

1. _____ to the invading organisms and the incomplete emptying of _____ compromise these protective mechanisms.

2. For the most part, factors predisposing clients to UTI result in _____ of the tract, _____ of the tract, or _____ in the function or structure of the tract.

3. Other contributing factors that were once believed to cause UTI, such as _____, panty hose and _____ are _____ considered significant in the development of UTI.

4. Most clients' symptoms can be reported as _____, _____, _____ in small amounts, _____, inability to empty the bladder, _____, cloudy urine…

5. Very simple changes in _____, _____, and _____ can make a huge difference in the clients' rate of re-infection.

书网融合……

微课1　　微课2　　微课3　　自测题

PPT

📖 **OBJECTIVES**

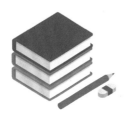

When you have completed Unit 6, you will be able to

⊙ understand and identify professional terms related to hypertension.

⊙ communicate with the doctor about some typical symptoms properly.

⊙ skim the passage for main idea.

⊙ describe the symptoms, the causes and the control of hypertension.

⊙ obtain more information about hypertension by listening to the lecture.

⊙ Master the structure "*the + comparative, the + comparative*".

📖 **LEAD IN**

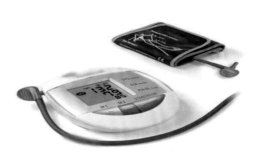

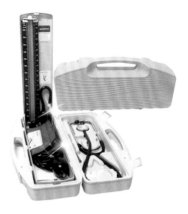

What are these devices?

What are they used for?

Do you know how to use them?

What does the number mean?

Classification of Blood Pressure for Adults

Category	Systolic, mmHg	Diastolic, mmHg
Hypotension	< 90	< 60
Desired	90 ~ 119	60 ~ 79
Prehypertension	120 ~ 139	80 ~ 89
Stage 1 hypertension	140 ~ 159	90 ~ 99
Stage 2 hypertension	160 ~ 179	100 ~ 109
Hypertensive emergency	≥ 180	≥ 110

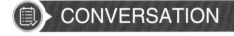 CONVERSATION

会话

John feels uncomfortable with his heart when he climbs steps, so he goes to the doctor.

Doctor: Have you ever fainted or had convulsions?

John: No.

Doctor: Do you ever feel dizzy, as if you or the room were moving?

John: No, never.

Doctor: Has a doctor ever told you that you had a heart murmur, or a heart attack, or high blood pressure?

John: No.

Doctor: Have you ever had any chest pain?

John: No.

Doctor: Do you have trouble climbing steps?

John: Well, yes. Climbing up the steps at home, I have to stop and catch my breath.

Doctor: About how many steps can you make before you have to stop?

John: Oh, ten or twelve, maybe.

Doctor: Have you mentioned this to a doctor before? Did he or she say anything about it?

John: Three years ago I went to the local hospital for a swimming certificate. They told me I had hypertension.

Doctor: Have you ever had swollen ankles?

John: Not that I can remember.

Doctor: What kind of treatment have you had in the past?

John: I took "reserpine" occasionally.

Doctor: Let me take your blood pressure.

Doctor: It's 150 over 95. That's moderately high. I would like you to do a urinalysis, blood urea nitrogen test，chest X-ray and an electrocardiogram examination.

Doctor：You should have a comprehensive test，avoid nervous tension or stress，and give up smoking and alcohol. In addition，I'll give you some medicine.

Doctor：Come back again next week for the results and another check of your blood pressure.

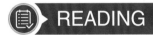 READING

Hypertension

Pre – reading

What is hypertension?

What are the symptoms of hypertension?

Is male or female more likely to get hypertension?

While – reading

Understanding Blood Pressure 微课1

You probably remember the routine from your last physical exam：A nurse wraps a cuff around your upper arm，pumps the cuff full of air，and then lets the air out slowly while listening through astethoscope or watching a machine. [1]

Every time the human heart beats，it pumps blood to the whole body through the arteries. Blood pressure is the force of blood pushing up against the blood vessel walls. The higher the pressure the harder the heart has to pump. [2] The normal level for blood pressure is below 120/80，where 120 represents the systolic measurement（peak pressure in the arteries）and 80 represents the diastolic measurement（minimum pressure in the arteries）. Blood pressure between 120/80 and 139/89 is called pre-hypertension（to denote increased risk of hypertension），and a blood pressure of 140/90 or above is considered hypertension.

What Is Hypertension?

Hypertension，also referred to as high blood pressure，is a condition in which the arteries have persistently elevated blood pressure. [3] Hypertension may be classified as essential or secondary. Essential hypertension is the term for high blood pressure with an unknown cause. It accounts for about 95% of cases. Secondary hypertension is the term for high blood pressure with a known direct cause，such as kidney disease，tumors，or birth control pills.

Hypertension can lead to coronary heart disease, heart failure, stroke, kidney failure, as well as other problems related to health.

Symptoms 🇪 微课2

There is no guarantee that a person with hypertension will present any symptoms of the condition.[4] About 33% of people and immunosuppressive actually do not know that they have high blood pressure, and this ignorance can last for years. For this reason, it is advisable to undergo periodic blood pressure screenings even when no symptoms are present.

Extremely high blood pressure may lead to some symptoms, however, and these include:

⊙ Severe headaches

⊙ Fatigue or confusion

⊙ Dizziness

⊙ Nausea

⊙ Problems with vision

⊙ Chest pains

⊙ Breathing problems

⊙ Irregular heartbeat

⊙ Blood in the urine

What Are the Causes?

Many prescription and over-the-counter drugs can cause or exacerbate hypertension. For example, corticosteroids and immunosuppressive drugs increase blood pressure in most solid-organ transplant recipients. Tobacco products (cigarettes, cigars, smokeless tobacco) contain nicotine, which temporarily increases blood pressure (for about thirty minutes or less). The blood pressure of smokers should be rechecked after thirty minutes if initial readings are high. This does not appear to be a direct relationship between caffeine and chronic hypertension, even acute (rapid but brief) increase in blood pressure.[5] This may be due to the fact that tolerance to caffeine develops rapidly.

Chronic overuse of alcohol is a potentially reversible cause of hypertension. Five percent of hypertension is due to alcohol consumption and 30 to 60 percent of alcoholics have it.

Diet and Hypertension 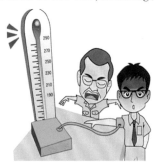 微课 3

Sodium intake has been a primary target for hypertension control though it is only ranked fourth as a lifestyle factor associated with hypertension. About 50 percent of individuals appear to be "sodium sensitive". This means that excessive sodium intake tends to increase blood pressure in these groups of people, and they do not appear to excrete excessive amount of salt via the kidneys.

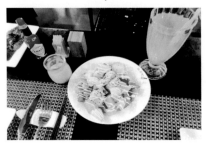

Sodium-sensitive individuals include elderly and obese individuals as well as African Americans. There are a number of ways to limit sodium in the diet, including:

⊙ do not use salt at the table

⊙ check food labels for sodium content

⊙ choose unprocessed foods

⊙ limit processed meats and cheeses

⊙ limit pickled meats and vegetables

⊙ limit salty snacks

⊙ limit intake of soy sauce, BBQ sauce, and

other condiments and foods that may be high in sodium.

Notes

1. A nurse wraps a cuff around your upper arm, pumps the cuff full of air, and then lets the air out slowly while listening through a stethoscope or watching a machine.

并列谓语 wraps, pumps 和 lets 保持形式上的一致。"while listening …or watching…" 为省略句。省略了 she is. 多出现省略（Ellipse）现象的时间状语从句引导词有 "when, while, before, after, till, until, once"。

省略遵循原则：当状语从句的主语与主句的主语一致时，可以省略状语从句的主语和系动词 be。如：（a）When（she was）very young, she began to learn to play the piano.（b）Before leaving, turn off all the lights.

2. The higher the pressure the harder the heart has to pump.

"the ＋比较级，the ＋比较级" 表示 "越…，就越…."。如：The more, the better.

该结构的完整表达方式为"the ＋比较级（＋主语）（＋谓语），the ＋比较级（＋主语）（＋谓语）"。如：The busier he is，the happier he will be.

主语谓语的省略主要体现在：①主、从句中的谓语动词是系动词 be，而且主语为非代词时，此时 be 常常省略。如：The higher the tree（is），the stronger the wind（is）.②主、从句的主语和谓语动词在叙述的场合有默契，可酌情省略。如：The more（you know），the more dangerous（it will be）.

3. Hypertension，also referred to as high blood pressure，is a condition in which the arteries have persistently elevated blood pressure.

明确区分三个短语"refer…to…"，"refer to"，"refer to…as"。

①refer A to B　把 A 提交给 B，把 A 归功于 B

When I registered high blood pressure，Doctor Brown referred me to Doctor Green，who is a specialist in hypertension.

②refer to… 查阅，参考；涉及；提及

a）If you want to know his telephone number，you may refer to the telephone directory.

b）Please don't refer to his past again.

c）These books refer to Asian problems.

③refer to A as B　把 A 称为 B

People refer to him as a living Lei Feng.

　＝He is referred to as a living Lei Feng.

原句中的 referred to as 即为过去分词作后置定语，也可以写为非限制性定语从句"which is referred to as high blood pressure"。英语中遵循从简的原则，所以能用过去分词等非谓语形式表达的就避免用从句的形式表达。

4. There is no guarantee that a person with hypertension will present any symptoms of the condition.

句式 There is no guarantee that…意为"…并无保证"。

5. There does not appear to be a direct relationship between caffeine and chronic hypertension，even though caffeine intake can cause an acute（rapid but brief）increase in blood pressure.

句型"There appears to be ＋主语"中的"appear"作为系动词，很多时候句型中的"to be"可以省略，翻译为"看起来、似乎……"。如：

A：It's too difficult，is there no other way?

B：There appears to be no alternative.

此类句型还有 There seems to be…看起来…，There used to be…曾经有……，There happens to be…碰巧有……，There ought to be…应该有……，There continues to be…依旧……等。例如：There used to be a printing house here 20 years ago.

Glossary

Word	English definition	Example
wrap *v.*	wrap sth. （up）（in sth.）to cover sth. completely in paper or other material IDM be wrapped up in sth. /sb	He spent the evening wrapping up the Christmas presents
cuff *n.*	something（as a part of a sleeve or glove）encircling the wrist	The blood pressure cuff and my sleeve cuff both tickle my arm
persistent *adj.*	determined to do sth. despite difficulties continuing for a long period of time without interruption	How do you deal with persistent salesmen who won't take no for an answer His cough grew more persistent until it never stopped
elevated *adj.*	1. high in rank 2. having a high moral or intellectual level 3. higher than the area around; above the level of the ground 4. higher than normal v. elevate adj. elevating（making people think about serious and interesting subjects） n. elevation n. elevator	When a patient's fever or blood pressure is elevated, treatment might be prescribed
essential *adj.*	completely necessary; extremely important	Experience is essential for this job
guarantee *n.*	a firm promise that you will do something or that something will happen	The doctor would give no guarantee that the treatment could stop the cancer
undergo *v.*	to experience something, especially a change or something unpleasant	Some children undergo a complete transformation when they become teenagers
periodic *adj.*	occurring or appearing at regular intervals	She was troubled by the periodic attacks of dizziness
exacerbate *v.*	to make something worse, especially a disease or problem	The symptoms may be exacerbated by certain drugs
transplant *v.*	to perform a medical operation in which an organ or other part that has been removed from the body of one person is put it into the body of another person	Surgeons have successfully transplanted a liver into a four-year-old boy
intake *n.*	the amount of food, drink, that you take into your body	Your intake of alcohol should not exceed two units per day
reversible *adj.*	1.（of clothes, materials）that can be turned inside out and worn or used with either side showing 2.（of a process, an action or a disease）that can be changed so that something returns to its original state or situation	Heart disease is reversible in some cases, according to a study published last summer
excrete *v.*	to pass solid or liquid waste matter from the body	Calcium is excreted in the urine and stools
pickle *v.*	To preserve food（vegetables, etc）in vinegar or salt water	My mother used to pickle cabbages
condiment *n.*	A substance such as tomato sauce or soya sauce that is used to give flavor to food	Most restaurants put condiments on the table so customers can add them to food as they wish

Word	English definition	Chinese definition
hypertension *n.*	blood pressure that is higher than is normal	高血压
stethoscope *n.*	an instrument that a doctor uses to listen to somebody's heart beat and respiration	听诊器
systolic *adj.*	systole：the part of the heart's rhythm when the heart pumps blood adj. systolic	心脏收缩的
diastolic *adj.*	diastole：the stage of the heart's rhythm when its muscles relax and the heart fills with blood adj. diastolic	心脏舒张的
tumor *n.*	a mass of cells growing in or on a part of the body where they should not，usually causing medical problems	瘤；肿瘤；肿块
coronary *adj.*	Surrounding like a crown（especially of the blood vessels surrounding the heart）	冠状动脉或静脉的
stroke *n.*	Sudden attack of illness in the brain that can cause loss of the power to move，speak clearly，etc.	中风
kidney *n.*	Either of a pair of organs in the body that remove waste products from the blood and produce urine	肾；肾脏
nicotine *n.*	a poisonous substance in tobacco that people become addicted to，so that it is difficult to stop smoking	尼古丁；烟碱
sodium *n.*	a chemical element，a soft silver-white metal that is found naturally only in compounds，such as salt	钠
corticosteroid *n.*	a steroid hormone produced by the adrenal cortex or synthesized	皮质类甾醇
immunosuppressive *adj.*	of or relating to a substance that lowers the body's normal immune response and induces immunosuppression	免疫抑制的
consumption *n.*	Using up of food，energy，resources，etc. Tuberculosis of the lungs	消耗；肺病

Post – reading

A1. True/False/Not Given Questions.

Refer to the passage and look at the statements below. Write

True　　　　if the statement agrees with the writer；

False　　　　if the statement does not agree with the writer；

NOT GIVEN if there is no information about this in the passage.

1. The human heart pumps blood to the whole body through the arteries.

2. A blood pressure of 120/80 or above is considered hypertension.

3. Essential hypertension，which occupies about 95% of cases，is caused by unknown

reasons.

4. Aboutone third of people actually do not know that they have high blood pressure.

5. The blood pressure of smokers should be rechecked after 30 minutes if initial readings are high.

6. The first target to control hypertension is to control sodium intake.

A2. Scan and complete the sentences.

1. A nurse _____ around your upper arm, pumps the cuff full of air, and then lets the air out slowly while listening through a stethoscope or watching a machine.

2. Blood pressure is the force of blood _____ the blood vessel walls.

3. Hypertension may be classified as _____ or _____ .

4. For this reason, it is advisable to _____ even when no symptoms are present.

5. This may be due to the fact that _____ develops rapidly.

B1. Choose the appropriate words and fill in the blanks with their correct forms.

| persist | undergo | reversible | elevate |
| essential | transplant | guarantee | wrap |

1. His cough grew more _____ until it never stopped.

2. Most authorities agree that play is an _____ part of a child's development.

3. The rapid rise in share prices helped _____ earnings last year.

4. Harry had carefully bought and _____ presents for Mark to give them.

5. Old jets _____ the process of modernization.

6. Good genes are no _____ of success.

7. Recognizing that something is _____ , makes it easier to take the leap.

8. He had a liver _____ in 2009.

B2. Match according to the explanations.

Word	Explanation
a. hypertension	
b. systolic	
c. aneurysm	iii. a class of chemicals that includes the steroid hormones that are produced in the adrenal cortex of vertebrates, and synthetic analogues of these hormones
d. diastolic	iv. a localized, blood-filled balloon-like bulge in the wall of a blood vessel
e. corticosteroid	v. it occurs when cells divide and grow excessively in the body
f. tumor	vi. a chronic medical condition in which the blood pressure in the arteries is elevated

B3. Guess the meaning from prefix and suffix.

hyper –	hypo –
hypertension – _____	hypotension – _____

cortico – 皮，皮质，皮层

corticoadrenal _____	corticoautonomic _____

C1. Multiple choice

1. The longer she waited, _____ she became.

A. the most impatient B. more impatient

C. the least impatient D. the more impatient

2. As far as I am concerned, education is about learning and the more you learn,

_____ .

A. the more for life are you equipped

B. the more equipped for life you are

C. the more life you are equipped for

D. you are equipped the more for life

3. _____ he comes, _____ I shall be.

A. The sooner; the happy B. The sooner; the happier

C. The sooner; happier D. Sooner; happier

4. _____ , the more it makes them cry.

A. The better the book they like B. The better they like the book

C. They like the book better D. They like the better the book

5. _____ , the more you eat.

A. The heavier are you B. The heavier you are

C. You the heavier D. You are the heavier

6. The earlier you _____ there, the less money it _____ .

A. get; will cost B. will get; will cost

C. get; cost D. will get; cost

C2. Multiple choice

1. Generally speaking, _____ according to directions, the drug has no side effect.

A. when taking B. when taken

C. when to take D. when to be taken

2. When _____ , the museum will be open to the public next year.

A. completed B. completing

C. being completed D. to be completed

3. The research is so designed that once _____ nothing can be done to change it.

A. begins   B. having begun

C. beginning   D. begun

4. While building a tunnel through the mountain, _____.

    A. an underground lake was discovered

    B. there was an underground lake discovered

    C. a lake was discovered underground

    D. the workers discovered an underground lake

C3. Rewrite the sentences according to the requirements.

C3 – 1   Write the phrases with elisions

1. While I was at college, I began to know him, a strange but able student.

    _____, I began to know him, a strange but able student.

2. You should let us know the result as soon as it is possible.

    You should let us know the result _____.

3. They are building a new plant while they are expanding the old one.

    They are building a new plant _____.

C3 – 2 Write the complete clause

1. While reading the newspaper, grandpa nodded from time to time.

    _____, grandpa nodded from time to time.

2. Don't come in until asked to.

    Don't come in _____.

3. Once a worker, Pang Long now becomes a famous singer.

    _____, Pang Long becomes a famous singer.

C4. Translation

1. 当被提问时，她一个字也说不出。(ellipse sentence)

2. 你练习的越多，理解的就越透彻。(the + comparative, the + comparative)

3. 那些在办公室工作的人被称为"白领工人"。(refer to … as)

4. 并不保证那些选上的一定会成为艺术家。(guarantee)

5. 看来这是毫无疑问的了。(there appears to be)

听力

LISTENING

Part A   Listen and answer the questions

1. What is the lecture about?

2. How many major classes of drugs combat hypertension?

3. Do many hypertension patients take only one type of drug?

4. Is he using or thinking about using non-prescription home remedy?

5. Who will also provide more information?

Part B　Complete the sentences

1. Diuretic lowers blood pressure by helping the _____ eliminate _____ and _____, _____ food from the body……. And the experts agree when diuretics _____ another drug, they can help their second drug work _____.

2. The next type of drug, a Vasodilator, actually relax the muscles on the _____ causing them to dilate and allow blood _____. As a result, the heart doesn't have to _____ and blood pressure _____.

3. A third type of drug, Alpha-blockers, also were to relax _____. They block the action of _____ in the body that normally causes the blood vessels to _____ or become narrower.

4. _____ are another class of drugs that were primary but we do see amounts of blood pump out of the heart.

5. Next are medicines that stop the production of the hormone and your tension too. These drugs are called _____. ACE stands for angiotensin-converting _____ …… The most common side effect is _____.

6. Finally, Calcium channel blockers _____ Calcium from _____ the cells of the heart and blood vessel walls……Consequently, we do see the calcium lower the pressure by _____ the blood vessels. It also decreases _____. When the heart pumps _____, the blood pressure is lowered.

书网融合……

微课1　　微课2　　微课3　　自测题

PPT

Unit 7　Angina

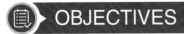

OBJECTIVES

When you have completed Unit 7, you will be able to

⊙ understand the meaning of the affixes "anti/ant –" and "– sclerosis".

⊙ master the preposition in sentences, such as "to, of …".

⊙ skim the passage for main idea.

⊙ describe the basic symptoms, the types and the causes of angina.

⊙ talk about the relationship between diet, hypertension and angina.

⊙ obtain helpful information about angina by listening to the lecture.

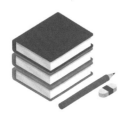

LEAD IN

Test your medical IQ

Q1: If you have a heart attack, you also have heart disease.

　　A. True　　　　　　　　　　B. False

Q2: Sudden cardiac arrest means that the heart…

　　A. stops beating

　　B. beats dangerously slow

　　C. has a circle of beating and stopping

　　D. skips beats

Q3: Symptoms of heart disease can include …

　　A. dizziness, weakness, arm pain, pressure in the chest

　　B. heart palpitations, shortness of breath, weakness

　　C. no symptoms at all

D. all of the above

Q4：Risks for heart disease include _____ .

A. high blood pressure and high cholesterol

B. smoking

C. lack of exercise

D. all of the above

Q5：The term "heart failure" means the heart has stopped working.

A. True　　　　　　　　　　B. False

Q6：The medical term for chest pain is _____ .

A. angina

B. There is no medical term for chest pain

C. flutter

D. arrhythmia

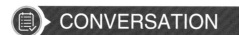 CONVERSATION

会话

On Saturday, Catherine held a party at home. Most of her friends came and had a wonderful night; however, her father seemed to be a little out of sorts. The next day, Catherine mentioned this to her brother Jack：

Catherine： Dad was really bad-tempered last night. That's just not like him. He used to like meeting my friends.

Jack： Well, I'm afraid they came at rather awkward time.

Catherine： What do you mean?

Jack： Well, I wasn't going to tell you, but Dad hasn't feeling very well lately.

Catherine： Has he seen the doctor?

Jack： Yes, he had a check-up last month. The doctor says he may have to go to the hospital.

Catherine： Oh no! What is it, exactly?

Jack： They are not sure. But they think it may be his heart.

Catherine： Oh, perhaps I ought to stay here. I'll tell the others to go ahead without me.

Jack： No, there's no point in that. It's not likely to be so serious. And, Catherine? Please don't say anything to Dad about this.

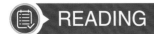 **READING**

Angina

Pre – reading

Have you ever met a person who has heart disease?

What is angina?

How is it treated?

While – reading

What Is Angina?

Angina, or angina pectoris, is chest pain, discomfort, or tightness that occurs when an area of the heart muscle is receiving decreased blood oxygen supply. It is not a disease itself, but rather a symptom of coronary artery disease, the most common type of heart disease.[1] The lack of oxygen rich blood to the heart is usually a result of narrower coronary arteries due to plaque buildup, a condition called atherosclerosis.[2] Narrow arteries increase the risk of pain, coronary artery disease, heart attack, and death.

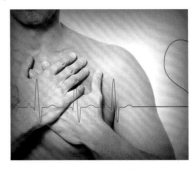

Types of Angina

Angina may manifest itself in the form of an angina attack, pain or discomfort in the chest that typically lasts from 1 to 15 minutes. The condition is classified by the pattern of attacks into stable, unstable, and variant angina.

Stable (or chronic) angina is brought on when the heart is working harder than usual, such as during exercise. It has a regular pattern and can be predicted to happen over months or even years. Symptoms are relieved by rest or medication.

Unstable angina does not follow a regular pattern. It can occur when at rest and is considered less common and more serious, as it is not relieved by rest or medicine.

Variant (Prinzmetal's) angina and microvascular (smallest vessels) angina are rare and can occur at rest without any underlying coronary artery disease. It is relieved by medicine.

Symptoms

Angina is usually felt as a squeezing, pressure, heaviness, tightening, burning or aching across the chest, usually starting behind the breastbone. This pain often spreads to the neck, jaw, arms, shoulders, throat, back, or even the teeth. Patients may also complain of symptoms that include indigestion, heartburn, weakness, sweating, nausea, cramping, and shortness of breath.

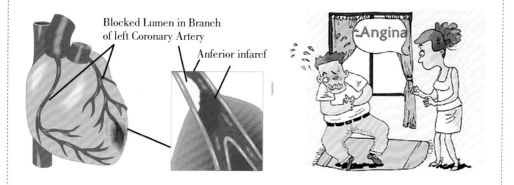

Blocked Lumen in Branch of left Coronary Artery

Anferior infarcf

Causes

Angina is most frequently the result of underlying coronary artery disease. The coronary arteries supply the heart with oxygen rich blood.[3] When cholesterol aggregate on the artery wall and hard plaques form, the artery narrows. It is increasingly difficult for oxygen rich blood to reach the heart muscle as these arteries become too narrow.[4]

In addition, damage to the arteries from other factors (such as smoking) can cause plaque to build up where the arteries are damaged. These plaques narrow the arteries or may break off and form blood clots that block the arteries.

The actual angina attacks are the result of this reduced oxygen supply to the heart. Physical exertion is a common trigger for stable angina, as the heart demands more oxygen than it receives in order to work harder. In addition, severe emotional stress, a heavy meal, exposure to extreme temperatures, and smoking may trigger angina.

Diet and Angina

Angina treatments aim to reduce pain, prevent symptoms, and prevent or lower the risk of heart attack. Medicines, lifestyle changes, and medical procedures may all be employed depending on the type of angina and the severity of symptoms.

Lifestyle changes recommended to treat angina include: stopping smoking, controlling weight, regularly checking cholesterol levels, resting and slowing down, avoiding large meals, learning how to handle or avoid stress, eating fruits, vegetables, whole grains, low-fat or no-fat diary products, and lean meat and fish. [5]

Medicines called nitrates (like nitroglycerin) are most often prescribed for angina. Nitrates prevent or reduce the intensity of angina attacks by relaxing and widening blood vessels. Other medicines such as beta blockers, calcium channel blockers, ACE inhibitors, oral anti-platelet medicines, anticoagulants, and high blood pressure medications may also be prescribed to treat angina. These medicines are designed to lower blood pressure and cholesterol levels, slow the heart rate, relax blood vessels, reduce strain on the heart, and prevent blood clots from forming.

In some cases, surgical procedures are necessary to treat angina. A heart specialist may recommend an angioplasty — a procedure where a small balloon is used to widen the narrowed arteries in the heart. Coronary artery bypass grafting is another common procedure; this is surgery where the narrowed arteries in the heart are bypassed using a healthy artery or vein from another part of the body.

Notes

1. It is not a disease itself, but rather a symptom of coronary artery disease, the most common type of heart disease.

句中……not……but……结构的意思为"不是……而是……"。连接两个并列的名词、形容词、副词、短语或分句等。例如：The meal is not for one, but for many to enjoy. "rather"用于语气的强调，可以翻译为"……. 不是……，而更（像）是…….."。如：Some argue that standardized tests do not indicate a student's academic skill but rather the ability to memorize and use a set of test taking tricks.

2. The lack of oxygen rich blood to the heart is usually a result of narrower coronary arteries due to plaque buildup, a condition called atherosclerosis.

此句中介词值得关注，如"the lack of, the blood to the heart, a result of, due to"中的介词 of 和 to。本文诸多介词及介词搭配出现，如：……manifest itself in the form of……; …… is classified by the pattern of attacks into……充分展示了介词虽小，作用奇大。"the blood to the heart"为介词 to 基本用法中"属于，归于"之意。如：the key to the house, the answer to the question。

3. The coronary arteries supply the heart with oxygen rich blood.

句中"supply A with B"为"动词 + 介词"短语，意为"为 A 提供 B"。如：The government supplies citizens with gas and electricity. 还可以用"supply B to A"来表达相同意思。如上句可以写为："The government supplies gas and electricity to citizens"。

4. It is increasingly difficult for oxygen rich blood to reach the heart muscle as these arteries become too narrow.

句式 It is difficult for sb. to do sth. 意为"对某人来说做什么事情是困难的"。如：It is difficult for us to finish the task. 该句中形容词 difficult 用来描述不定式 to do sth. 因此，可写为 to do sth. is difficult. 若将 difficult 换为形容词"nice"，其后介词也要改为 of，整个句式改为：It is nice of sb. to do sth. 此时 nice 用来描述 sb 而不是不定式，因此可写为 Sb. is nice to do sth. 综上所述，It is ＋adj. ＋of/for sb. ＋to do sth.

当 adj. 为品质形容词，如 kind，good，nice，right，wrong，clever，careless，polite，foolish 等，且句子可改写为 Sb. is ＋adj. to do sth. 即选用句式 It is ＋adj. ＋of sb. to do sth.

当 adj. 为描述事物形容词，如 difficult，easy，hard，important，dangerous，(im)possible 等，且句子可改写为 to do sth. is ＋adj. 即选用句式 It is ＋adj. ＋for sb. to do sth.

5. Lifestyle changes recommended to treat angina include：stopping smoking, controlling weight, regularly checking cholesterol levels, resting and slowing down, avoiding large meals, learning how to handle or avoid stress, eating fruits, vegetables, whole grains, low-fat or no-fat diary products, and lean meat and fish.

此句中关注两点。第一，该段落为一句话，其中核心句子为"Lifestyle changes recommended to treat angina include……."而"recommended to treat angina"为后置定语，所以主谓结构就剩下"lifestyle changes include……"。医药类文章中很多长句出现，看清哪是句子主要结构，哪是修饰，更有助于理解句子，把握文章内容。第二，句中并列成分的列举，保持结构的一致。如：stopping……，controlling……，checking……，resting……，avoiding……，learning……，eating……

Glossary

Word	English definition	Example
discomfort *n.*	a feeling of slight pain or of being physically uncomfortable	You will experience some minor discomfort during the treatment
manifest *v.*	manifest itself (in sth.)：to appear or become noticeable	The symptoms of the disease manifested themselves ten days later
variant *n. /adj.*	a thing that is a slightly different form or type of something else	This game is a variant of baseball variant forms of spelling
predict *v.*	to say that something will happen in the future	Nobody could predict the future
relieve *v.*	to remove or reduce an unpleasant feeling or pain	Aspirin relieved the pain of the migraine (headache)
underlying *adj.*	Important in a situation but not always easily noticed or stated clearly	Unemployment may be an underlying cause of the rising crime rate

续表

Word	English definition	Example
squeeze *v.*	topress something firmly, especially with your fingers	He squeezed her hand and smiled at her
aggregate *v.*	to put together different items, amounts into a single group or total	The scores were aggregated with the first round totals to decide the winner
trigger *v.*	to make something happen suddenly	Nuts can trigger off a violent allergic reaction
exposure *n.*	the state of being in a place or situation where there is no protection from something harmful or unpleasant	Continuous exposure to sound above 80 decibels could be harmful
employ *v.*	touse something such as a skill, method for a particular purpose	The police had to employ force to enter the building
severity *n.*	something hard to endure	The new drug lessens the severity of pneumonia episodes
handle *v.*	to be in charge of, act on, or dispose of	To tell the truth, I don't know if I can handle the job
lean *adj.*	to be lacking excess flesh	After one month training for the basketball team, the parents barely recognized their lean son
graft *v.*	placethe organ or part of a body of a donor into the body of a recipient	I am having a skin graft on my arm soon

Word	English definition	Chinese definition
angina *n.*	a heart condition marked by paroxysms of chest pain due to reduced oxygen to the heart	心绞痛
plaque *n.*	(pathology) a small abnormal patch on or inside the body	斑块
atherosclerosis *n.*	a stage of arteriosclerosis involving fatty deposits inside the arterial walls	动脉粥样硬化
indigestion *n.*	a disorder of digestive function characterized by discomfort or heartburn or nausea	消化不良 ⓔ 微课 1
cramp *n.*	cramp is a sudden strong pain caused by a muscle suddenly contracting	痛性痉挛；抽筋
cholesterol *n.*	an animal sterol that is normally synthesized by the liver; the most abundant steroid in animal tissues	胆固醇
clot *n.*	coalesce or unite in a mass	血块
nitrate *n.*	any compound containing the nitrate group (such as a salt or ester of nitric acid)	硝酸盐
anticoagulants *n.*	a class of drugs that work to prevent the coagulation (clotting) of blood	抗凝［血］剂
angioplasty *n.*	an operation to repair a damaged blood vessel or unblock a coronary artery	血管成形术
bypass *n.*	a conductor having low resistance in parallel with another device to divert a fraction of the current	导管

Post – reading

A1. True/False/Not Given Questions.

Refer to the passage and look at the statements below. Write

True   if the statement agrees with the writer;

False   if the statement does not agree with the writer;

NOT GIVEN if there is no information about this in the passage.

1. Angina is a kind of disease that occurs when an area of the heart muscle is receiving decreased blood oxygen supply.

2. There are two types of Angina.

3. Patients with angina may have indigestion and nausea.

4. When cholesterol aggregates on the artery wall and hard plaques form, the artery becomes cramped.

5. Surgical medical procedures are necessary in most cases to treat angina.

A2. Scan and complete the sentences.

1. Angina is a symptom of _____, the most common type of heart disease.

2. Stable angina has a _____ and can be _____ to happen over months or even years.

3. Angina is usually felt as a _____, _____, _____, etc.

4. Angina can be caused by _____, _____, _____ .

5. Nitrates _____ or _____ the intensity of angina attacks by _____ and _____ blood vessels.

B1. Choose the appropriate words and fill in the blanks with their correct forms.

> manifest   predict   relieve   squeeze
>
> underlying   severity   exposure   trigger

1. It was a _____ in the car with five of them.

2. Weather forecasts _____ more hot weather, gusty winds and lightning strikes.

3. I think that the _____ problems are education, unemployment and bad housing.

4. Smiling and laughing have actually been shown to _____ tension and stress.

5. Unresolved or unacknowledged fears can _____ sleepwalking.

6. _____ to lead is known to damage the brains of young children

7. Their frustration and anger will _____ itself in crying and screaming.

8. Several drugs are used to lessen the _____ of the symptoms.

B2. Match according to the explanations.

Word	Explanation
a. angina	i.
b. plaque	ii.
c. atherosclerosis	iii. any compound containing the nitrate group (such as a salt or ester of nitric acid)
d. cholesterol	iv.
e. anticoagulants	v.
f. nitrate	vi. medicine that prevents or retards the clotting of blood

B3. Guess meaning from prefix and suffix.

atherosclerosis

athero – _____

– sclerosis _____, dentinal sclerosis: _____

anticoagulants

anti/ant – _____

antibiotics: _____

anti – diarrhea action: _____

anticancer: _____

antibody: _____

C1. Multiplechoice

1. _____ the science demonstration, the whole exhibition was well designed.

    A. Except   B. Apart   C. Beside   D. With the exception of

2. In his speech he _____ to the great help the school received from the government.

A. expressed   B. explained   C. referred   D. whispered

3. You'd better _____ your books after reading them.

A. put up   B. put on   C. put down   D. put away

4. Let's learn to use the problem we are facing _____ a stepping-stone to future success.

A. to   B. for   C. as   D. by

5. Fred entered without knocking and, very out of breath, sank _____ a chair.

A. on   B. off   C. into   D. to

6. The nurses in that hospital are very good _____ the patients there.

A. at   B. for   C. to   D. with

7. Let's dance _____ the music.

A. with   B. from   C. to   D. by

C2. Multiple choice

1. Most of the artists _____ to the party were from South Africa.

A. invited

B. to invite

C. being invited

D. had been invited

2. The computer center, _____ last year, is very popular among the students in this school.

A. open

B. opening

C. having opened

D. opened

3. Cleaning women in big cities usually get _____ by the hour.

A. pay   B. paying   C. paid   D. to pay

4. —How do you deal with the disagreement between the company and the customers?

—The key _____ the problem is to meet the demand _____ by the customers.

A. to solving; making

B. to solving; made

C. to solve; making

D. to be solved; made

5. Don't use words, expressions, or phrases _____ only to people with specific knowledge.

A. being known

B. having been known

C. to be known

D. known

C3. Rewrite the sentences into simple sentences.

1. The glass which was broken by my son has been swept away.

2. The Town Hall which was completed in the 1800's was the most distinguished building at that time.

3. We will go to visit the bridge which was built hundreds of years ago.

4. The books which were written by Lu Xun are popular.

5. Is this the book which is recommended by the teacher?

C4. Translation

1. 我们要去参观那座建于几百年前的桥。

2. 他失败了，不是因为他不聪明而是因为他工作不努力。（not…but…）

3. 学校为我们提供了整洁的环境。（supply…with…）

4. 对于孩子来说，单独过马路是非常危险的。

5. 由于疏忽大意造成的错误可能带来严重的后果。（due to）

LISTENING

听力

Part A　Listen and answer the questions.

1. What does Arnold suffer from?

2. Why does Angina need to be treated well?

3. What can help to decrease the blockage of blood?

4. What kind of medications does Arnold take? How many medications does he take every day?

5. How can the doctor identify where the blockage is located?

Part B　Complete the sentences.

1. Dr. Stern：It means that you are _____ .

2. The heart is a powerful pump made up of muscles. Like all muscles, it needs _____ and _____ .

3. The pain of angina is caused by _____ .

4. Dr. Stern：We think that _____ may play a role in this, _____ may play a role in this, as well as _____ .

5. In the treatment of angina, what I am trying to do is to _____ .

6. If these factors don't help the angina, then we do have _____ .

7. When the balloon is in position, the doctors carefully began to _____ . They do several inflations _____ . They can use pressure _____ atmospheric pressure.

书网融合……

微课1　　　　微课2　　　　微课3　　　　自测题

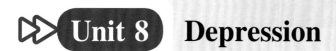 **Unit 8 Depression**

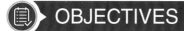 **OBJECTIVES**

When you have completed Unit 8, you will be able to

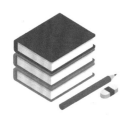

⊙ understand and identify expressions related to depression.

⊙ communicate with the doctor about some typical symptoms properly.

⊙ skim the passage for main idea.

⊙ describe the definition, the types and self help remedies of the depression.

⊙ master the usage of *"that"* in attributive clause.

⊙ obtain more causes about depression disorder by listening to the lecture.

LEAD IN

When you have been in blue for a period of time, you may doubt you are suffering from depression. The following is a list of depression symptoms. Please check your conditions with the list and don't describe yourself in depression unless they last for more than two weeks.

⊙ persistently sad, anxious, angry, irritable, or "empty" mood

⊙ feelings of hopelessness or pessimism

⊙ feelings of worthlessness, helplessness, or excessive guilt

⊙ loss of interest in hobbies and activities that were once enjoyed

⊙ social isolation, meaning the sufferer avoids interactions with family or friends

⊙ insomnia, early morning awakening, or oversleeping

⊙ decreased appetite and/or weight loss, or overeating and/or weight gain

⊙ fatigue, decreased energy, being "slowed down"

⊙ crying spells

⊙ thoughts of death or suicide, suicide attempts

⊙ restlessness, irritability

⊙ difficulty concentrating, remembering, or making decisions

⊙ persistent physical symptoms that do not respond to treatment, such as headaches, digestive disorders, and/or chronic pain

CONVERSATION

A patient suffering from insomnia is having a conversation with the doctor.

Doctor：Good morning. What seems to be the problem?

Patient：I've been suffering from nervousness recently, which makes me feel rather upset. I feel very tired and exhausted.

Doctor：Can you tell me something more in detail?

Patient：I have difficulty in falling asleep, and I'm a very light sleeper. When I wake up, my heart beats very fast and I'm sweating heavily.

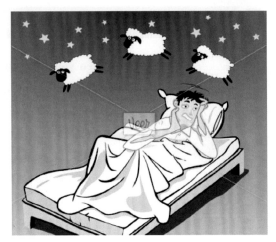

Doctor：Anything else?

Patient：I always have nightmares. All of this has influenced my study.

Doctor：How long has this been going on?

Patient：Three months, ever since the preparation of additional sports examination. You know, I'm not good at sports, and my parents expect me to be admitted to the key senior high school.

Doctor：So you are under great pressure, and you don't want to let your parents down.

Patient：Exactly.

Doctor：I think you are suffering from insomnia. Let me take your blood pressure; you look anemic. [after taking blood pressure] Well, there is nothing serious. Have you taken any medicine?

Patient：I tried some sleeping pills, but they didn't work. What should I do now?

Doctor：I think you need more rest. Don't fatigue yourself unnecessarily. Take it easy and adjust your mental condition.

Patient：I know. But sometimes it is easier said than done.

Doctor：The most important thing is to overcome your nervousness. You should always look at the good side of things. Your parents will understand you and be always on your side.

Patient：I suppose so.

Doctor：As long as you have tried your best, there is nothing to regret.

Patient：Well, what you've said makes me feel much better now, Doctor. I think I can sleep well tonight. Thank you very much.

Activity

Try to answer the questions based on the conversation.

1. What's wrong with this patient?

A: He is suffering from heart attack.

B: He is suffering from high blood pressure.

C: He is suffering from insomnia.

D: He is suffering from psychosis.

2. What are his symptoms?

A: He feels weary and upset.

B: He perspires a lot sometimes.

C: He is sleeping poorly and always has nightmares.

D: All of the above.

3. How long has he had this problem?

A: Two months.

B: Three months.

C: Ever since he attended the key senior high school.

D: Ever since his parents forced him to study.

4. What diagnostic tools did the doctor use to examine him?

A: Blood pressure meter.

B: Electrocardiogram

C: Blood glucose monitor.

D: Cardiopulmonary Resuscitation. （CPR）

5. What did the doctor prescribe for him?

A: Some sleeping pills.

B: More exercises.

C: Trying to get along wellwith his parents.

D: Overcoming his nervousness and becoming adjusted.

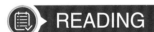 READING

Depression

Pre – reading

What is the definition of a depressive disorder?

What are the three types of depression?

Can you think of some other remedies?

While – reading

What Is a Depressive Disorder?

A depressive disorder is a syndrome (group of symptoms) that reflects a sad and/or irritable mood exceeding normal sadness or grief. More specifically, the sadness of depression is characterized by a greater intensity and duration and by more severe symptoms and functional disabilities than is normal.

Depressive signs and symptoms are characterized not only bynegative thoughts, moods, and behaviors but also by specific changes in bodily functions[1]. For example, crying spells, body aches, low energy or libido, as well as problems with eating, weight, or sleeping.

Depressive disorders are a huge public health problem, due to its affecting millions of people. Facts about depression include that approximately 10% of adults, up to 8% of teens, and 2% of preteen children experience some kind of depressive disorder.

Types of Depression

Type 1 Major Depression

Major depression is characterized by a combination of symptoms that last for at least two weeks in a row, including sad and/or irritable moods, that interfere with the ability to work, sleep, eat, and enjoy once-pleasurable activities. Difficulties in sleeping or eating can take the form of

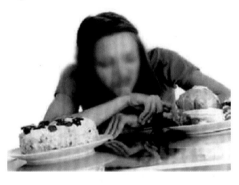

excessiveness or insufficiency of either behavior.[2] Disabling episodes of depression can occur once, twice, or several times in a lifetime.

Type 2 Dysthymia

Dysthymia is a less severe but usually more long-lasting type of depression compared to major depression. It involves chronic symptoms that do not disable but yet prevent the affected person from functioning at "full steam" or from feeling good.[3] Sometimes, people with dysthymia also ex-

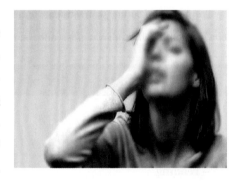

perience episodes of major depression. This combination of the two types of depression often is referred to as double-depression.

Type 3 Bipolar disorder[4]

Another type of depression is bipolar disorder, which encompasses a group of mood disorders that were formerly called manic-depressive illness or manic depression. These conditions show a particular pattern of inheritance. Not nearly as common as the other types of depressive disorders, bipolar disorders involve cycles of mood that include at least one episode of mania and may include episodes of depression as well.[5] Bipolar disorders are often chronic and recurring. Sometimes, the mood switches are dramatic and rapid, but most often they are gradual. Mania often affects thinking, judgment, and social behavior in ways that cause serious problems and embarrassment.

Self – help Home Remedies

⊙ Eat healthy foods. The frequent lack of adequate nutrients and presence of excessive fats, sugars and sodium in fast foods can further sap the energy of depression sufferers.

⊙ Many may find that folate and vitamin D food supplements help improve their mood.

⊙ Make time to get enough rest to physically promote improvement in your mood.

⊙ Express your feelings.

⊙ Do not set difficult goals for yourself or take on a great deal of responsibility.

⊙ Break large tasks into small ones, set some priorities, and do what you can when you can.

⊙ Do not expect too much too soon as this will only increase feelings of failure.

⊙ Try to be with other people.

⊙ Participate in activities that may make you feel better.

⊙ You might try exercising, going to a movie or a ball game, or participating in religious or social activities.

⊙ Do not make major life decisions, such as changing jobs or getting married or divorced without consulting others who know you well. It is advisable to postpone important decisions until your depression has lifted.

Notes

1. Depressive signs and symptoms arecharacterized not only by…

句中 characterized by…是“动词 + 介词”短语，意为“以…为特征”。

eg：The giraffe is characterized by its very long neck.

2. Difficulties in sleeping or eating can take the form of excessiveness or insufficiency of either behavior

句中 take the form of…是“动词 + 名词 + 介词”短语，意为“表现为…的形式”。

eg：Our class took the form of group discussion and summary.

3．It involves chronic symptoms that do not disable but yet prevent the affected person from functioning at "full steam" or from feeling good.

本句中由 that 引导的定语从句 " do not disable but yet prevent the affected person from functioning at 'full steam' or from feeling good" 修饰了先行词 "chronic symptoms"，that 多指物，有时也指人，在定语从句中作主语或宾语。其中 prevent sb. /sth. （from doing sth.）意为 "阻止或妨碍某人/某物（做某事）" eg：The earthquake prevented people from sleeping safely at home last night.

4．Bipolar disorder 双相忧郁症；这一型的忧郁症患者时而充满精力，可以连续工作几天几夜，极其兴奋，脾气暴躁，感官异常灵敏；随之而来的是连续几个星期的低潮期，患者表现乏力，没精神，对什么都提不起兴趣，可以赖在床上一天不动，厌食……大部分双相忧郁症患者脑部运作方式和精神分裂类似，以分散无连续性的思维为主要症状之一，换言之，他们都不具备逻辑思维的能力。

5．Not nearly as common as the other types of depressive disorders, bipolar disorders involve cycles of mood that include at least one episode of mania and may include episodes of depression as well.

"not nearly" 是一个副词，表示 "远不及，完全不" 的意思。这个复杂句的主语是 "bipolar disorders"，谓语是 "involve"，宾语是 "cycles of mood"。后面的部分 "that include at least one episode of mania and may include episodes of depression as well" 作为一个定语从句（attributive clause）来修饰前面的先行词 "cycles of mood"。全句的中文翻译如下 "双相忧郁症远不及其他类型的抑郁症普遍，它包括的情绪周期中最起码含有一个狂躁期，也可能含有多个一般性抑郁阶段。"

Glossary

Word	English definition	Example
exceed v.	be greater in scope or size than some standard	His knowledge of history exceeds mine
duration n.	the period of time during which something continues	The duration of the movie is 110 minutes
negative adj.	marked by features of hostility, withdrawal, or pessimism that hinder or oppose constructive treatment or development	Now I am afraid of getting a negative response from the judge since I made a slight mistake
spell n.	a period of indeterminate length (usually short) marked by some action or condition	It looks as if we were in for a cold spell
approximately adv.	about; estimated to be	There were approximately fifty people there at the graduation ceremony for the tiny class
in a row prep.	continuously	This is the third Sunday in a row that it's rained
interfere with v.	come between so as to be hindrance or obstacle	Constant interruptions interfere with my work

Word	English definition	Example
episode *n.*	a happening that is distinctive in a series of related e-vents	Attending the lecture series with the famous scientist was an episode in my life I won't ever forget
encompass *v.*	include as part of something broader;	The general arts at the university encompass a wide range of subjects
manic *adj.*	affected with or marked by frenzy or mania uncontrolled by reason	The performers had a manic energy and enthusiasm
inheritance *n.*	(genetic) attributes acquired via biological heredity from the parents	Her blue eyes were a paternal inheritance
recurring *adj.* recur *v.*	repeating happen again; happen repeatedly	There is the source of the recurring pestilence
remedy n.	treatment, medicine, etc that cures or relieves a disease or pain; countering or removing sth. undesirable	He found a remedy for his grief in constant hard work
sap *v.*	deplete, exhaust	The negative criticism sapped his determination
priority *n.*	status established in order of importance or urgency	Improving the plight of teachers is indeed a priority item
postpone *v.*	hold back to a later time; delay	She didn't postpone her departure even though a severe weather warning was in effect
Word	English definition	Chinese definition
syndrome *n.*	a pattern of symptoms indicative of some disease	证候群；综合征
libido *n.*	(psychoanalysis) a Freudian term for sexual urge or desire	性欲，欲望
dysthymia *n.*	mild chronic depression;	精神抑郁症
folate *n.*	a B vitamin that is essential for cell growth and reproduction	叶酸

Post – reading

A1. Yes/No/Not Given Questions

Refer to the passage and look at the statements below. Write

YES　　　　　if the statement agrees with the writer;

NO　　　　　if the statement does not agree with the writer;

NOT GIVEN　if there is no information about this in the passage.

1. A depressive disorder is a syndrome that reflects a sad and/or irritable mood exceeding normal sadness or grief.

2. It's almost impossible for preteens to suffer from depressive disorders.

3. It's difficult to predict how many incidences of disabling episodes of depression may occur in a lifetime.

4. The combination of dysthymia and major depression is referred to as double-depression.

5. Havingadequate nutrients can help people evade depression.

A2.　Answer the following questions.

1. What are the bodily changes if one suffers from depression?

2. Why are depressive disorders a huge public health problem?

3. Should we suspect his having a major depression when a person is having too much sleeping?

4. What is a double depression?

5. Among all the self-help home remedies, which are particularly helpful for you when you are not so happy?

B1.　Choose appropriate words and fill in the blanks with their correct forms.

inheritance	negative	priority	postpone
interfere	exceed	recur	encompass

1. The fine shall not ＿＿＿＿＿＿ $ 300.

2. The dream ＿＿＿＿＿＿ throughout her life.

3. Don't ＿＿＿＿＿＿ in matters that do not concern you!

4. The answer to my request was in the ＿＿＿＿＿＿.

5. The atmosphere ＿＿＿＿＿＿ the earth.

6. Half of the people who ＿＿＿＿＿＿ the gene express it.

7. At the worst, the storm will make us ＿＿＿＿＿＿ the trip.

8. Safety has high ＿＿＿＿＿＿ in factories.

B2.　Match the words with their synonyms.

1. inheritance	a) preference
2. negative	b) include, involve
3. priority	c) meddle, disturb
4. postpone	d) heritage, birthright
5. interfere	e) delay
6. exceed	f) surpass
7. recur	g) dcnying
8. encompass	h) repeat

B3. Study the following affix, decide its meaning and match more words that end with the same affix with their Chinese equivalents.

B3 −1 interfere

The word "interfere" contains an affix "inter". What does it mean?

1. interpose	a）国际的
2. international	b）人际间的
3. intersect	c）置于，介入
4. interpersonal	d）横断

B3 −2 dysthymia

1. dysfunction	a）呼吸困难
2. dysphagia	b）吞咽困难
3. dyspnea	c）功能紊乱
4. dysarthria	d）构音困难

C1. Combine the two simple sentences into a complex sentence with attributive clauses.

eg：*This is the most important word. We have learned it today.*

This is the most important word that we have learned today.

1. They threw out the computer. It ever worked properly.

2. This is the lion. It has been ill recently.

3. The building is an exhibition center. It is on the other side of the river.

4. I don't like the man. He is quarrelling with his colleagues.

5. Have you found the key? It was lost last week.

C2. Translate the following sentences into Chinese and pay attention to the attributive clauses.

1. Endangered languages are languages that are slowly disappearing because of technology and the desire for cultures to assimilate.

2. Addiction is a brain disease that changes a person's neurochemistry.

3. Overpopulation and fresh water shortage are two thorny problems that people are confronted with today.

4. Traditional schools offer cultural and sports activities that the home-schooled children will miss out on.

5. The people that you met on campus yesterday are from England.

C3. Translation

1. 日常的运动和合理的饮食是人们保持健康的最好方法。

2. 请把那幅画盖起来，别让雨水打湿了它。（prevent…from…）

3. 有人看到了你昨天丢失的车。

4. 这次会议是以成果展示和分组讨论的形式进行的。（take the form of…）

5. 这是我收到的最珍贵的礼物。

LISTENING

听力

Part A You are going to hear a science report on Teens, Television and Depression. Please first complete the sentences with the numbers you hear.

1. Thefindings were based on more than ＿＿＿＿＿ adolescents.

2. The survey began in ＿＿＿＿＿.

3. The survey reveals that the total media use reaches ＿＿＿＿＿ hours a day, among which the television watching was more than ＿＿＿＿＿ hours.

4. More than ＿＿＿＿＿ percent of the young man had signs of depression in ＿＿＿＿＿.

5. Doctor Primack says every extra hour of television meant an ＿＿＿＿＿ percent increase in the chances of developing signs of depression.

Part B Identify whether the following information is True or False based on your understanding of the listening material.

1. The study claims that the more teenagers there are watching TV, the more likely they are to develop depression.

2. The findings were based on more than four thousand adolescents.

3. Given the same amount of media use, young women were more likely than men to develop depression.

4. The study says that watching TV was the cause of depression because watching TV may take away time that might be used for social activities.

5. Sociologists from the University of Maryland find that the happier people are those who are more likely to be socially active, to read, to attend religious services and to vote.

书网融合……

微课1　　微课2　　微课3　　自测题

Unit 9　Alcoholism

PPT

LEAD IN

Amy Winehouse was an English singer-song writer who was the first British female to win five Grammys. BBC has called her "the preeminent vocal talent of her generation". However, at the age of 28, she died unexpectedly of alcohol poisoning on 23 July 2011.

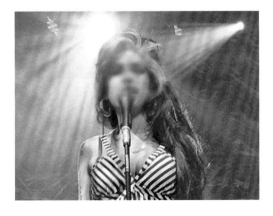

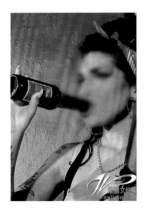

Do you like Amy's songs?

Do you feel pity for her sudden death?

What should be blamed for it?

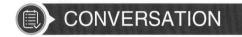 **CONVERSATION**

会话

A patient addicted to alcohol is having a conversation with his doctor. Please list diseases related to alcohol use.

Doctor：Good morning. You look much more sober today. Not drinking alcohol can really improve your state of mind.

Patient：You're right, doctor. But you know I still cannot resist the temptation of wine. Is drinking really so harmful?

Doctor：Sure. Researchers have linked alcohol consumption to more than 60 diseases. Heavy drinking can cause the number of oxygen-carrying red blood cells to be abnormally low. This condition, known as anemia, can trigger a host of symptoms, including fatigue, shortness of breath, and lightheadedness.

Patient：Yeah! That sounds pretty serious!

Doctor：But if you develop into a heavy drinker, especially a binge drinker, it makes platelets more likely to clump together into blood clots. Heart attack or stroke will easily happen.

Patient：Oh, that's a bit scary. I should be more careful with the amount and the frequency of using alcohol.

Doctor：Yes, you should. I know your family has a history of gout. Although gout is largely hereditary, alcohol plays a role in aggravating it.

Patient：Oh, I'm vulnerable to gout. I would never want to have that kind of painful condition like my mom. I should control my desire for alcohol.

Doctor：Apart from gout, heavy drinking and bingeing, in particular —— can cause blood pressure to rise. Over time, this effect can become chronic. High blood pressure can lead to many other health problems, including kidney disease, heart disease, and stroke.

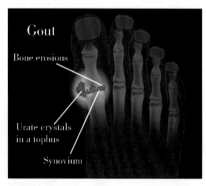

Patient：It seems overuse of alcohol can trigger any disease you can imagine.

Doctor：That's not the worst. Heavy drinking can cause a form of nerve damage known as alcoholic neuropathy, which can produce a painful pins-and-needles feeling in the extremities, as well as muscle weakness, incontinence, constipation, and other problems.

Patient：I now fully understand the damages alcohol can bring to body and mind. I will try my best to curb my desire for alcohol and I promise I won't have more than one cup a day.

Doctor：I already see your progress. Keep it up and I'm sure you can get rid of alcohol abuse.

Patient：Thank you, doctor. I won't achieve present state without your constant warning and encouragement. I will always bear your words in mind.

Doctor：I believe you mean what you say. Remember to visit me next Monday.

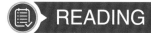 READING

Alcoholism

Pre – reading

Do you think alcoholism is a disease?

Can you name some of the symptoms of alcoholism?

Does alcohol affect men and women differently?

While – reading

What Is Alcoholism?

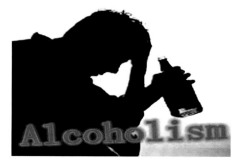

Alcoholism, formerly called alcohol dependence or alcohol addiction, is the more severe end of the alcohol use disorder spectrum. It is a destructive pattern of alcohol use that includes tolerance to or withdrawal from the substance, using more alcohol or using it for longer than planned, and trouble reducing its use or inability to use it in moderation. [1] Other potential symptoms include spending an inordinate amount of time getting, using, or recovering from the use of alcohol, compromised functioning, and/or continuing to use alcohol despite an awareness of the detrimental effects it is having on one's life.

Alcoholism is appropriately considered a disease rather than a weakness of character or chosen pattern of bad behavior. It is the third most common mental illness, affecting more than 14 million people in the United States.

Symptoms and Signs

Signs that indicate a person is intoxicated include the smell of alcohol on their breath or skin, glazed or bloodshot eyes, the person being unusually passive or argumentative, and/or a deterioration in the person's appearance or hygiene. [2] Other physical symptoms of the state of being drunk include flushed skin. Cognitively, the person may experience decreased ability to pay attention and a propensity toward memory loss.

Alcohol, especially when consumed in excess, can affect teens, women, men, and the elderly quite differently. Women and the elderly tend to have higher blood concentrations of alcohol compared to men and younger individuals who drink the same amount.[3] Alcoholic women are more at risk for developing cirrhosis of the liver and heart and nerve damage at a faster rate than alcohol-dependent men. Interestingly, men and women seem to have similar learning and memory problems as the result of excessive alcohol intake, but again, women tend to develop those problems twice as fast as men.[4]

The Stages of Alcohol Use Disorder

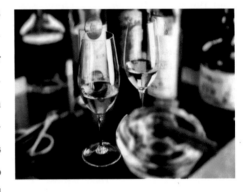

Five stages of alcohol use disorders have been identified. The first stage is described as having access to alcohol rather than use of alcohol. In that stage, minimizing the risk factors that make a person more vulnerable to using alcohol are an issue. The second stage of alcohol use ranges from experimentation or occasional use to regular weekly use of alcohol. The third stage is characterized by individuals further increasing the frequency of alcohol use and/or using the substance on a regular basis. This stage may also include either buying or stealing to get alcohol. In the fourth stage of alcohol use, users have established regular alcohol consumption, have become preoccupied with getting intoxicated and have developed problems in their social, educational, vocational, or family life. The final and most serious fifth stage of alcohol use is defined by the person only feeling normal when they are using alcohol. During this stage, risk-taking behaviors like stealing, engaging in physical fights, or driving while intoxicated increase, and they become most vulnerable to having suicidal thoughts.

The Treatment for Alcoholism

Prior to entering any inpatient or outpatient rehabilitation program for alcohol use disorder, the possibility that the person with this disorder could suffer from physical symptoms of alcohol withdrawal needs to be addressed.[5] People who have a pattern of extensive alcohol abuse are at risk for withdrawal symptoms like tremors, hallucinations, and even fatal seizures. Those individuals will need to enter a detoxification program that includes the use of close medical support, monitoring, and prescription of medications like chlordiazepoxide (Librium) or clonazepam (Klonopin) to help prevent and ease the symptoms of alcohol withdrawal.

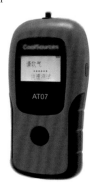

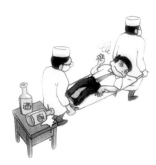

The approach to those who have experimented with alcohol should not be minimized by mental-health professionals, since infrequent use can progress to the more serious stages of alcohol use if not addressed. Therefore, professionals recommend that the alcohol-consuming individual be thoroughly educated about the effects and risks of alcohol, that fair but firm limits be set on the use of alcohol, and that the user be referred for brief counseling, a self-help group, and/or family support group. People who have progressed to the more advanced stages of alcoholism are typically treated intensively, using a combination of the medical, individual, and familial interventions.

Notes

1. It is a destructive pattern of alcohol use that includes tolerance to or withdrawal from the substance, using more alcohol or using it for longer than planned, and trouble reducing its use or inability to use it in moderation. 这是一个含有限制性定语从句的复杂句。主句为 "It is a destructive pattern of alcohol use," 意为 "这是一种破坏性的酒精饮用行为。" 后面紧跟的定语从句详细描述了 "这种破坏性的酒精饮用行为" 的三种表现，"包括沉迷于酒精或戒断酒精，比原定计划使用更多酒精或更长时间内饮酒，和控制饮酒量困难或无法做到适量饮酒。"

2. Signs that indicate a person is intoxicated include the smell of alcohol on their breath or skin, glazed or bloodshot eyes, the person being unusually passive or argumentative, and/or a deterioration in the person's appearance or hygiene. 这句话的主干部分是 "Signs… include …," 主语是 "signs"，谓语是 "include"，后面的都是宾语部分。

3. Women and the elderly tend to have higher blood concentrations of alcohol compared to men and younger individuals who drink the same amount.

句中 "who drink the same amount" 是关系代词 who 引导的定语从句，用以修饰 who

的先行词 "men and younger individuals"，who 在从句中用作主语。

4. Interestingly, men and women seem to have similar learning and memory problems as the result of excessive alcohol intake, but again, women tend to develop those problems twice as fast as men. 句中 tend to 意为 "趋向，偏重"，as…as… 意为 "像…一样…" 其结构为：as + adj. / adv. + as eg：as beautiful as flower.

5. Prior to entering any inpatient or outpatient rehabilitation program for alcohol use disorder, the possibility that the person with this disorder could suffer from physical symptoms of alcohol withdrawal needs to be addressed. 句中由关系代词 that 引导的定语从句 "that the person with this disorder could suffer from physical symptoms of alcohol withdrawal" 修饰限定了先行词 "the possibility".

suffer from 意为 "遭受…（病痛/折磨）"。

Glossary

Word	English definition	Example
moderation *n.*	quality of being moderate and avoiding extremes	The secret of health is moderation in all things
inordinate *adj.*	beyond normal limits	She had an inordinate fondness for junk food
compromise *v.*	settle by concession	They found it wiser to compromise with her
detrimental *adj.*	(sometimes followed by 'to') causing harm or injury	Lack of sleep is detrimental to one's health
intoxicate *v.*	make drunk (with alcoholic drinks)	Too much wine intoxicates people
glaze *v.*	(used of eyes) lacking liveliness	His eyes glazed over with boredom
argumentative *adj.*	given to or characterized by argument	He is an intelligent but argumentative child
deterioration *n.*	process of changing to an inferior state	I definitely felt a deterioration in vigor
identify *v.*	recognize as being; establish the identity of someone or something	The markings are so blurred that it is difficult to identify
vulnerable *adj.*	susceptible to criticism or persuasion or temptation	Young birds are very vulnerable to predators
range from…to … *v.*	Change or be different from one extremity to another	The room rate at this motel range from $30 to $50 per day
consume *v.*	eat immoderately; or drink something	I'm sure that Chinese people consume the largest amount of rice in the world
preoccupied *adj.*	having or showing excessive or compulsive concern with something;	Why is humanity so preoccupied with right and wrong
engage in *v.*	carry out or participate in an activity; be involved in	Is it wise to engage in active sports at your age
prior to *prep.*	earlier in time	Prior to his death, the criminal confessed everything to the police
rehabilitation *n.*	the treatment of physical disabilities by massage and electrotherapy and exercises	Drug rehabilitation is a long and painful process

Word	English definition	Example
minimize *v.*	make small or insignificant	Governments consider it prudent to minimize the risk
address *v.*	direct one's efforts towards something	The next meeting will address the problem of truancy
refer *v.*	send or direct for treatment, information, or a decision	They decided to refer this patient to a specialist

Word	English definition	Chinese definition
withdrawal *n.*	stop having a substance, normally this word goes together with symptoms	戒断（毒品、酒精等），常与"症状"连用，特指医学概念上的"戒断症状"
hygiene *n.*	a condition promoting sanitary practices	卫生，卫生学
cirrhosis *n.*	a chronic disease interfering with the normal functioning of the liver; the major cause is chronic alcoholism	硬化，肝硬化
tremor *n.*	shaking or trembling	颤抖
hallucination *n.*	illusory perception; a common symptom of severe mental disorder	幻觉
seizure *n.*	a sudden occurrence (or recurrence) of a disease	突然发作
detoxification *n.*	a treatment for addiction to drugs or alcohol intended to remove the physiological effects of the addictive substances	解毒，去毒作用
chlordiazepoxide *n.*	an antianxiety, sedative, hypnotic drug	甲氨二氮䓬, 利眠宁（安定药）
clonazepam *n.*	anticonvulsant	氯硝西泮（抗惊厥药）

Post – reading

A1. Yes/No/Not Given Questions

Refer to the passage and look at the statements below. Write

YES　　　　　　if the statement agrees with the writer;

NO　　　　　　if the statement does not agree with the writer;

NOT GIVEN　　if there is no information about this in the passage.

1. People who are addicted to alcoholism are not aware of the detrimental effects.

2. Alcoholism is a weakness of character or chosen pattern of bad behavior.

3. Women are more vulnerable to alcohol-related disease.

4. Regular weekly use of alcohol belongs to the third stage of alcoholism.

5. Mental-health professionals should give more attention to people who are at the beginning stages of alcohol use.

A2. Five stages of alcohol use disorders have been identified. Please match the stages with their appropriate features.

Stages	Features
The First Stage	Be preoccupied with getting intoxicated; develop problems in various aspects of life
The Second Stage	Having access to alcohol
The Third Stage	Feeling normal only when using alcohol; increased risk-taking behaviors.
The Fourth Stage	Occasional use or regular weekly use of alcohol
The Fifth Stage	Increased frequency, drink on a regular basis

B1. Choose the appropriate words and fill in the blanks with their correct forms.

> withdrawal   moderation   compromise   hygiene
>
> vulnerable   deterioration   preoccupied   minimize

1. We should try our best to _____ risks inconstructing a bridge.

2. A civilized citizen should contribute his/her efforts to public _____ .

3. Even if you only smoke in _____ this is a good time to stop.

4. _____ from heroin is never easy for anyone.

5. His knees were his _____ spot.

6. I cannot relinquish the thought of furthering my education abroad; I'm _____ as a result.

7. After a two-week negotiation, the two sides finally _____ over the hard-fought text.

8. He had trouble with bone _____ and walked with a cane.

B2. Match the words with their synonyms.

1. compromise	a) susceptible
2. detrimental	b) inebriate
3. consume	c) eat/ drink
4. identify	d) damaging
5. intoxicate	e) diminish, reduce
6. deteriorate	f) break down
7. vulnerable	g) concession
8. minimize	h) recognize

B3. Study the following affix, decide its meaning and match more words that end with the same affix with their Chinese equivalents.

B3 – 1 cirrhosis

The word "cirrhosis" contains an affix "osis". What does it mean?

1. thrombosis	a）矽肺病
2. atherosclerosis	b）动脉粥样硬化
3. tuberculosis	c）血栓
4. volcanokoniosis	d）结核

B3 – 2 detoxification

The above word "detoxification" contains "de". What does it mean?

1. dehydrate	a）解码
2. deactivate	b）灭活
3. decode	c）脱色
4. decolor	d）脱水

C1. Translate the following sentences into Chinese, pay attention to the underlined part.

1. These decorations can't compare with each other, they are different styles.

2. No one received the notification prior to today's date.

3. The boy plays either basketball or computer games in his spare time.

4. I think I will walk around in the field rather than stay at home.

5. His physical condition was particularly bad as a result of drinking to excess.

C2. In terms of structure, there are four types of sentences. They are simple sentences, compound sentences, complex sentences, and compound-complex sentences. Analyze the following sentences and decide which type they belong to.

1. We often study Chinese history on Friday afternoon.

2. The boy who offered me his seat is called Tom.

3. There is a chair in this room, isn't there?

4. My brother and I go to school at half pastsix in the morning and come back home at seven in the evening.

5. He is in Class One, and I am in Class Two.

6. He was fond of drawing when he was yet a child.

7. Neither has he changed his mind, nor will he do so.

8. What he said at the meeting is very important, isn't it?

9. The farmer is showing the boy how to plant a tree.

10. Both Tom and Jack enjoy country music.

C3. Translation

1. 我们应该多从事对社会有意义和有用的事。（engage in）

2. 显然，他们付出了和我们一样多的努力。（as…as…）

3. 他们正遭受着健康问题的困扰并担心着辐射带来的其他麻烦。（suffer from…）

4. 高血压患者的年龄从十几岁的孩子到几十岁的老人不等。（range from…to…）

5. 我认识那个因酒驾而被警察带走的女孩。

听力

LISTENING

You are going to hear a science report on *The Economic cost of Alcoholism*. Refer to the listening and look at the statements below. Write

True　　if the statement agrees with the listening material.

False　　if the statement does not agree with the listening material.

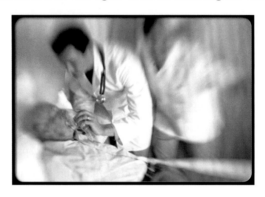

1. The biggest costs of excessive alcohol drinking come from a loss of worker productivity.

2. The annual cost of excessive alcohol drinking is ＄220 billion.

3. Alcohol-related costs don't include property damage from road accidents.

4. Many people with a drinking problem have lower-paying jobs.

5. It is a personal tragedy if people die of alcohol-attributable conditions.

6. Other nations do not have problems with the "harmful use of alcohol".

7. The economic costs in different countries vary.

8. British singer Amy Winehouse died as a result of drinking too much alcohol.

书网融合……

微课1　　　　微课2　　　　微课3　　　　自测题

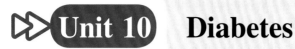 **Unit 10** **Diabetes**

PPT

OBJECTIVES

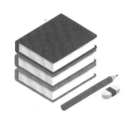

When you have completed Unit 10, you will be able to

⊙ understand and identify professional terms related to diabetes.

⊙ communicate with a physician how to avoid diabetes.

⊙ skim the passage for main idea.

⊙ describe the basic symptoms, the types, and the causes of diabetes.

⊙ obtain information about diabetes by listening to the lecture.

⊙ master the use of "*are being done*".

LEAD IN

Diabetes Quiz Game

Q1	Q2	Q3	Q4	Q5	Q6	Q7	Q8

Q1: Diabetes is defined best as···

A. A metabolic disease characterized by low blood sugar

B. A metabolic disease characterized by high blood sugar

C. A family of blood infections

D. None of the above

Q2: Diabetes can be cured with diet, exercise, and medication.

A. True

B. False

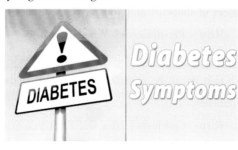

Q3: Which is not a symptom of diabetes?

A. Itchy skin   B. Thirst

C. Frequent urination   D. Muscle pain

Q4： If you have diabetes, you're more likely to get the flu.

    A. True   B. False

Q5： People with diabetes should not eat candy or other sugary foods.

    A. True   B. False

Q6： It's dangerous for women with diabetes to get pregnant.

    A. True   B. False

Q7： How much aerobic activity should most people with diabetes get each week?

    A. 60mins   B. 80mins

    C. 100mins   D. 150mins

Q8： Why should you wear comfortable shoes and sneakers?

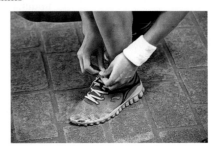

    A. To prevent DFAS (diabetic fallen arch syndrome)

    B. To prevent shin splints

    C. To prevent foot injuries

    D. None of the above

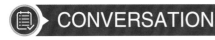 **CONVERSATION**

会话

Ritu goes to see his doctor after receiving the test report.

Ritu： Good morning, doctor!

Doctor： Good morning!

Ritu： Here is my test result.

Doctor： Er, the A1C is a little bit high.

Ritu： How high? What's normal? Does it matter? Is it serious?

Doctor： Take it easy! The problem is not that serious if you take good care of it. The normal A1C is below 5.7%, and your result is 6%. That means you are at high risk for the development of diabetes and you have pre-diabetes.

Ritu： Pre-diabetes? What's that?

Doctor： Pre-diabetes means your blood glucose level is higher than normal but not so high that it can be categorized as type 2 diabetes. It takes 10 years or less to develop into type 2 diabetes.

Ritu： Goodness! How did I get that?

Doctor： In most cases, overweight is the main cause of prediabetes and the older we are, the higher the risk will be.

Ritu： Oh, I am 47, and my BMI is 31. Definitely I've got both. Doctor, am I sure to get diabetes?

Doctor：Absolutely not. You can prevent this con-dition from developing into diabetes by changing to a healthy lifestyle that includes daily physical activities, maintaining a healthy weight and eating healthy foods.

Ritu：Would you please give me some tips?

Doctor：I'd love to. First, you must relax by sleeping for at least 6 to 8 hours. This will help your metabolic system to lose the extra weight and reduces the stress in your life. Second, it is good to exercise 30 minutes a day or 5 days a week to maintain healthy

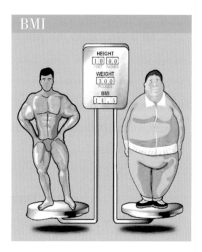

weight. Third, opt for healthy eating habits like low fat proteins such as fish, chicken, and vegetables like spinach, onions, tomatoes, mixed greens, broccoli and some fruits like cherries, apples and blueberries. Good food choices also include low-glycemic foods, organic foods, and foods with fatty acids. Finally, learn more information about nutrition and consult a physician if possible.

Ritu：Thank you very much. I'll obey the rules and take care of myself!

READING

Diabetes

Pre – reading

What is diabetes?

What are the symptoms of diabetes?

Does diabetes only occur in adults?

While – reading

What is Diabetes?

Diabetes means that your blood glucose, also called blood sugar, is too high. Glucose comes from the food you eat and is needed to fuel our bodies. [1] Glucose is also stored in our liver and muscles. Your blood always has some glucose in it because your body needs glucose for energy. But having too much glucose in your blood is not healthy.

An organ called the pancreas makes insulin. Insulin helps glucose get from your blood into your cells. Cells take the glucose and turn it into energy. If you have diabetes, the pancreas makes little or no insulin or your cells cannot use insulin very well. Glucose builds up in your blood and cannot get into your cells. If your blood glucose stays too high, it can damage many parts of the body such as the heart, eyes, kidneys, and nerves.

Are There Different Types of Diabetes?

Yes. There are three main types of diabetes. In type 1 diabetes, the cells in the pancreas that make insulin are destroyed. If you have type 1 diabetes, you need to get insulin from shots or a pump everyday. Most teens can learn to adjust the amount of insulin they take according to their physical activity and eating patterns. Type 1 used to be called "insulin dependent" or "juvenile" diabetes.

In type 2 diabetes, the pancreas still makes some insulin but cells cannot use it very well. If you have type 2 diabetes, you may need to take insulin or pills to help your body's supply of insulin work better. Type 2 used to be called "adult onset diabetes." Now more teens are getting type 2, especially if they are overweight.

Gestational diabetes is a type of diabetes that occurs when women are pregnant. Having it raises their risk for getting diabetes, mostly type 2, for the rest of their lives. It also raises their child's risk for being overweight and for getting type 2 diabetes.

Symptoms of Diabetes

Type 1 and Type 2 diabetes impede a person's carefree life. Symptoms like polydipsia (thirsty), polyuria (frequent urination), polyphagia (hunger), and excessive weight loss can be observed in a diabetic.[2] Desired blood sugar of human body should be between 70 ~ 110 mg/dl at fasting state. If blood sugar is less than 70 mg/dl, it is termed as *hypoglycemia* and if more than 110 mg /dl, it's *hyperglycemia*.

Diabetes is the primary reason for adult blindness, end-stage renal disease (ESRD), gangrene and amputations. When blood sugar level is constantly high it leads to kidney failure, cardiovascular problems and neuropathy. Patients with diabetes are 4 times more likely to have coronary heart disease and stroke.

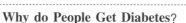

Why do People Get Diabetes?

Both genes and things like viruses and toxins may cause a person to get type 1 diabetes. Studies are being done to identify the causes of type 1 diabetes and to stop the process that destroys the pancreas.[3]

Researchers can now predict who is at risk for developing type 1 diabetes and in the future may be able to prevent or delay the onset of the disease.

Being overweight/obese increases the risk for type 2 diabetes.

It causes the body to release chemicals that can destabilize the body's cardiovascular and metabolic systems. The risk of developing type 2 diabetes is also greater as we get older. Experts are not completely sure why, but say that as we age we tend to put on weight and become less physically active. Some racial groups have a greater chance of getting diabetes-American Indians, Alaska Natives, African Americans, Hispanics/Latinos, Asian Americans, and Pacific Islanders. It is not true that eating too much sugar causes diabetes.

What Do I Need to Do to Take Care of My Diabetes?

The key to taking care of your diabetes is to keep your blood glucose as close to normal as possible.[4] The best way to do this is to:

⊙ Make healthy food choices

⊙ Eat the right amounts of food

⊙ Be active everyday

⊙ Stay at a healthy weight

⊙ Take your medicines and check your blood glucose as planned with your health care team

Your doctor will tell you what blood glucose level is right for you. Your goal is to keep your blood glucose as close to this level as you can. Your doctor or diabetes educator will teach you how to check your blood glucose with a glucose meter. It helps to know what affects your blood glucose level. Food, illness, and stress raise your blood glucose. Insulin or pills and being physically active lower your blood glucose. Carbohydrates, or carbs for short, are a good source of energy for our bodies. But if you eat too many carbs at one time, your blood glucose can get too high. Many foods contain carbs. Great carb choices include whole grain foods, nonfat or low-fat milk, and fresh fruits and vegetables. Eat more of them rather than white bread, whole milk, sweetened fruit drinks, regular soda, potato chips, sweets, and desserts.

Notes

1. Glucose comes from the food you eat and is needed to fuel our bodies.

"you eat" 为省略了 that 的定语从句，修饰 food。并列谓语由 and 连接，保持时态一致的同时，注意谓语动词的变化（comes 与 is needed 并列）。

2. Symptoms like polydipsia（thirst）, polyuria（frequent urination）,

polyphagia（hunger）, and excessive weight loss can be observed in a diabetic.

英语构词法（word formation）有多种，其中词缀构词法（affixation）最为常见。

affixation =（prefix）＋root ＋（suffix）

prefix	root	suffix	word
poly － : too any/much	－ dipso － : thirsty	－ ia：condition	polydipsia：a kind of condition that shows too much thirsty

3. Studies are being done to identify the causes of type 1 diabetes and to stop the process that destroys the pancreas.

"are being done" 为现在进行时的被动语态，表示现在正在被做的事情。其结构由现在进行时（am/is/are ＋Ving）和被动语态（be ＋ Vpp）整合而成：am/is/are ＋being ＋ Vpp

4. The key to taking care of your diabetes is to keep your blood glucose as close to normal as possible.

the key to doing

the key is to do sth

as close to normal as possible

Glossary

Word	English definition	Example
shot *n.*	injection or needle	The kid took a flu shot yesterday
juvenile *adj.*	connected with young people who are not yet adults	Even as a juvenile, Tom showed great responsibility, caring for his sick grandfather after school every day
onset *n.*	the beginning of something, especially something unpleasant	Many people dread the onset of disease, old age, and winter
Impede *v.*	(often passive, formal) hinder and hamper to delay or stop the progress of something	Work on the building was impeded by severe weather
excessive *adj.*	greater than what seems reasonable or appropriate	Excessive drinking can lead to stomach disorders
fast *v.*	to eat little or no food for a period of time, especially for religious or health reasons	Muslims fast during Ramadan

续表

Word	English definition	Example
predict *v.*	to foretell or forecast what something will happen in the future adj. predictable& predictive n. prediction	Nobody could predict the outcome of the experiment
destabilize *v.*	to undermine the security of a system; for example, physical body, or political government	Terrorist attacks were threatening to destabilize the government
pregnant *adj.*	carrying developing offspring within the body or being about to produce new life	Tina was pregnant with their first daughter

Word	English definition	Chinese definition
diabetic *adj.* &n.	a medical condition caused by a lack of INSULIN, which makes the patient produce a lot of URINE and fell very thirsty	糖尿病的，糖尿病患者
pancreas *n.*	an organ near the stomach that produces INSULIN and a liquid that helps the body to DIGEST food	胰脏
insulin *n.*	a chemical substance produced in the body that controls the amount of sugar in the blood	胰岛素
gestation *n.*	the time that the young of a person or an animal develops inside its mother's body until it is born	怀孕，酝酿
polydipsia *n.*	an excessive thirst (as in cases of diabetes or kidney dysfunction)	［医］烦渴
polyuria *n.*	renal disorder characterized by the production of large volumes of pale dilute urine; often associated with diabetes	［医］多尿（症）
polyphagia *n.*	an abnormal desire to consume excessive amounts of food, especial as the result of a neurological disorder	多食症
hypoglycemia *n.*	a condition characterized by abnormally low blood glucose (blood sugar) levels, usually less than 70 mg/dl	［医］血糖过低；低血糖症
hyperglycemia *n.*	the technical term for high blood glucose (blood sugar), which happens when the body has too little insulin or when the body can't use insulin properly	多糖症；多血糖症
end-stage renal disease *n.*	according to the American Kidney Fund, end stage renal disease (ESRD) is when the kidneys cease to function well enough to allow a person to live without a kidney transplant or dialysis	［医］终末期肾脏疾病
gangrene *n.*	the localized death of living cells (as from infection or the interruption of blood supply)	［医］坏疽，腐败
amputation *n.*	a surgical removal of all or part of a limb	［医］截肢
cardiovascular *adj.*	of, relating to, or involving the heart and the blood vessels	［医］心血管的
neuropathy *n.*	a disease or abnormality of the nervous system	神经病
coronary *n.*	of or relating to the heart	冠状动脉
carbohydrate *n.*	any of a group of organic compounds which contain only carbon, hydrogen, and oxygen, usually in the ratio $1:2:1$	碳水化合物
metabolic *adj.*	relating to the process in which food is changed into energy, new cells, and waste products in plants and animals	［生物学］新陈代谢的
kidney *n.*	either of two bean-shaped excretory organs that filter wastes (especially urea) from the blood and excrete them and water in urine	肾，肾脏

Post – reading

A1. Scan and complete the sentences.

1. Diabetes means your _____ is too high.

2. _____ , which is made by _____ , helps glucose get from your blood into your _____ .

3. If your blood glucose stays too high, it can damage many parts of the body such as the heart, eyes, _____ , and _____ .

4. Diabetes can be roughly categorized into _____ kinds: _____ , _____ , and _____ .

5. Diabetes may lead to many problems, such as _____ , _____ , _____ , _____ .

6. People who are easy to get type 2 are _____ , _____ , and _____ .

7. We can take care of our diabetes by _____ , _____ , _____ , _____ , _____ .

8. We'd better eat _____ rather than _____

_____　　　　_____

_____　　　　_____

A2. Read the passage and answer the following questions.

1. Where is the storage of glucose?

2. How many types of diabetes?

3. Whatare the symptoms of diabetes?

4. How do the patients take care of their diabetes?

B1. Choose the appropriate words and fill in the blanks with their correct forms.

> juvenile, onset, shot, impede,
> excessive, fast, predict, destabilize

1. So the meal that breaks your _____ should be healthy and wholesome.

2. Fallen rock is _____ the progress of rescue workers

3. A _____ delinquent is a person who is typically under the age of 18 and commits an act that otherwise would have been charged as a crime if they were an adult.

4. _____ dosage of this drug can result in injury to the liver.

5. At no time can the feed system _____ an otherwise stable ombustion process.

6. Earthquake _____ is still a young science.

7. Bilingualism even seems to delay the _____ of dementia in old age.

8. This is absolutely my favourite _____ .

B2. Write down the word that is mostly related to the picture.

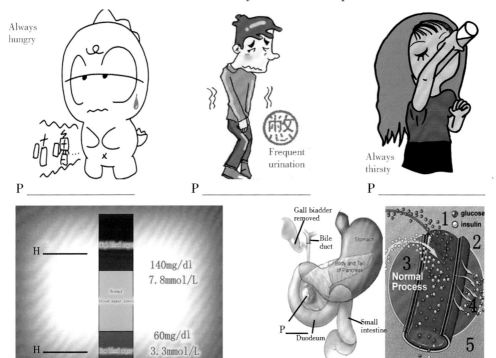

Always hungry

Frequent urination

Always thirsty

P _____   P _____   P _____

H _____   140mg/dl
7.8mmol/L

H _____   60mg/dl
3.3mmol/L

H _____   H _____   P _____

Step 1 Stomach converts food to G _____

Step 2 G _____ enters bloodstream

Step 3 G _____ produces sufficient i _____ but it is resistant to effective use

Step 4 G _____ unable to enter body effectively

Step 5 G _____ levels increase

B3. Match

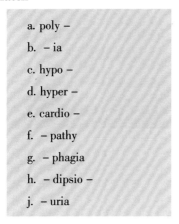

a. poly –   i. urine

b. – ia   ii. disease

c. hypo –   iii. drinking

d. hyper –   iv. eating

e. cardio –   v. condition of being ill

f. – pathy   vi. many, much

g. – phagia   vii. low

h. – dipsio –   viii. heart

j. – uria   ix. high

B4. Guess

Word	Meaning	Word	Meaning
dysuria（dys = bad or difficult）		hyperbaric	
cardiogram（gram = sth written with drawn）		pathology	
neuropathy		insomnia（somn = sleep）	
hypodermic（dermic = the skin）		autophagia	

C1. Multiple choice

1. I don't know what time it is now. My watch _____ .

    A. is repairing   B. has been repaired

    C. is being repaired   D. has repaired

2. It is said that pandas _____ in our country year after year.

    A. are being disappeared   B. are disappearing

    C. will be disappeared   D. will disappear

3. —I don't suppose the police know who did it.

    —Well，surprisingly they do. A man has been arrested and _____ now.

    A. has being questioned   B. is questioning

    C. has questioned   D. is being questioned

4. The camera you _____ now _____ to me.

    A. use；is belonged   B. are using；is belonged

    C. use；is belonging   D. are using；belongs

5. The bridge which _____ last year _____ really beautiful.

    A. was built；looks   B. was building；looks

    C. was built；is looked   D. was building；is looked

C2. Complete the sentences with the words given.

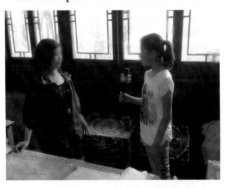

（Mary，interview）

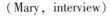

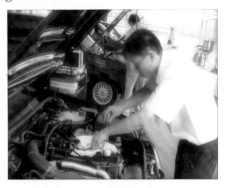

（my car，repair）

_____

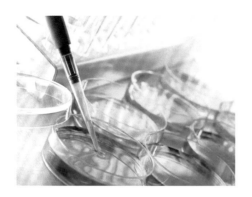

（the disease，study）

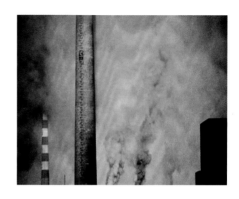

（our environment，pollute）

_____

_____

C3. Translation

1. 孩子们正受到良好的照顾。

2. 正在做什么试验？

3. 昨天我去逛了逛街，买了些书，Tom 还请我吃了一顿大餐。

4. 你认为保持健康体重的关键是什么？我觉得关键是有规律地运动。

5. 关键点都是尽可能保持身体最接近自然体温 37 摄氏度。

听力

LISTENING

Part A   Listen carefully and finish the following sentences with "True" or "False".

1. Organizers warn of a Diabetes epidemic affecting 264 million people worldwide.

2. World Diabetes Day falls on November fifteen.

3. Over time，diabetes can cause blindness，kidney disease and nerve damage.

4. Type 1 diabetes can be controlled through diet，exercise and treatment.

5. Doctor Kaufman says type 2 diabetes is spreading as more people rise out of poverty in developing countries.

Part B   Complete the sentences within NO MORE THAN THREE WORDS.

1. People with _____ have too much _____ , or sugar，in their blood.

2. The body changes food for energywith the help of _____ .

3. FRANCINE Kaufman："Children are in cars all day long，and they've got _____ outside their houses. They are eating more food，and more _____ food and getting

overweight. "

4. And people are getting on buses and going to office and not _____ being as _____ as they have been in the past.

5. The message of World Diabetes Day is that the disease is _____ and, in the case of type two diabetes, _____ .

书网融合······

e 微课1

e 微课2

e 微课3

自测题

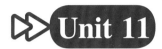 **Unit 11** **Hyperthyroidism**

PPT

OBJECTIVES

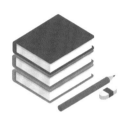

When you have completed Unit 11, you will be able to

⊙ understand and identify professional terms related to hyperthyroidism.

⊙ communicate with a physician about the hyperthyroidism.

⊙ skim the passage for main idea.

⊙ master the attributive clauses introduced by *which* and *in which*.

⊙ describe the basic symptoms and the causes of hyperthyroidism.

⊙ obtain the main information by listening to the report.

LEAD IN

What's wrong with them?

What kind of disease can cause these problems?

What are the typical symptoms?

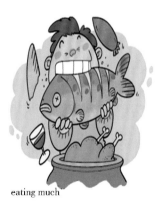

eating much

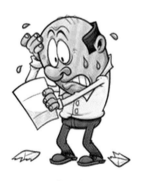

Sweating

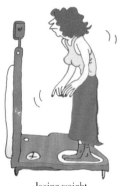

losing weight

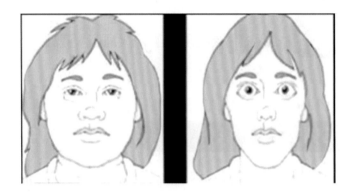

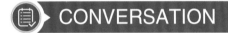 CONVERSATION

会话

Luis went to see his doctor as he did not feel good this morning.

Luis：Good morning，Doctor Lee.

Lee：Good morning! What's the matter?

Luis：I've got angry easily and I feel quite uncomfortable with my heart for the past two months.

Lee：Have you ever felt this way before?

Luis：Actually，this has been happening for the past 2 months only.

Lee：Have you lost any weight recently?

Luis：Yes，I have，in spite of eating more than usual，I still managed to lose 10 pounds in 2 months.

Lee：Have you been sleeping well?

Luis：Lately I've been suffering from insomnia.

Lee：Have you been sweating as much as before this?

Luis：My sweating has increased notably. I just can't stand warm weather at all.

Lee：All right，would you please get undressed now? Let me examine you. Now，swallow，please.

Luis：Thank you，doctor.

Lee：There are some tests you'll have to get done and we'll see you in one week. At that time we'll start on a definite therapy for your condition.

Luis：Thanks again，but please tell me what's wrong?

Lee：I suspect that you might have hyperthyroidism. Take this paper to the office，and the nurse will arrange a time for you to have some thyroid function testing.

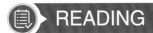 READING

Hyperthyroidism

Pre – reading

What is hyperthyroidism?

What are the symptoms of hyperthyroidism?

Are men or women more likely to get hyperthyroidism?

While – reading

What Is Hyperthyroidism?

Hyperthyroidism, or overactive thyroid disease, means your thyroid gland makes and releases too much thyroid hormone. The thyroid gland is located in the front of your neck, just below your Adam's apple[1]. It makes hormones that control your metabolism. Metabolism is the pace of your body's processes and includes things like your heart rate and how quickly you burn calories.

The neck

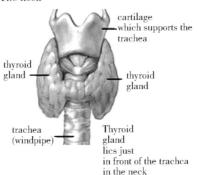

cartilage which supports the trachea

thyroid gland

thyroid gland

trachea (windpipe)

Thyroid gland lies just in front of the trachea in the neck

What Are the Symptoms of Hyperthyroidism?

Hyperthyroidism usually begins slowly, so its symptoms can be mistaken for stress or other health problems.[2] It can cause a variety of symptoms, including:

⊙ nervousness, anxiety or irritability

⊙ weight loss

⊙ fatigue

⊙ increased sensitivity to heat

⊙ increased appetite

⊙ increased perspiration

⊙ changes in bowel patterns

⊙ muscle weakness

⊙ difficulty sleeping

⊙ rapid heartbeat, irregular heartbeat or pounding of the heart

⊙ tremors (trembling of the hands and fingers)

⊙ changes in menstrual patterns (usually lighter flow, less frequent periods) in women

⊙ an enlarged thyroid gland (called a goiter), which can appear as a swelling at the base of the neck

Older adults may have subtle symptoms, such as increased heart rate, increased perspiration and a tendency to become moretired during normal activities. If your hyperthyroidism is caused by Graves' disease, you may also have Graves' ophthalmopathy, a disorder that affects your eyes. These symptoms may show up before, after or at the same time as your symptoms of hyperthyroidism. In Graves' ophthalmopathy, the muscles behind the eyes swell and push the eyeballs forward. Often, the eyeballs will actually bulge out of their normal position. The front surfaces of the eyeballs become dry, red and swollen. You may notice excessive tearing or discomfort in your eyes, sensitivity to light, blurry or double vision, and less eye movement.

What Causes Hyperthyroidism?

In more than 70% of cases, hyperthyroidism is caused by an autoimmune disorder called Graves' disease. Normally, antibodies produced by the immune system help protect the body against viruses, bacteria and other foreign substances. An autoimmune disease is when your immune system produces antibodies that attack your body's tissues and/or organs.

Two other common causes for hyperthyroidism include:

⊙ Hyperfunctioning thyroid nodules. One or more nodules or lumps in the thyroid grow and increase their activity so that they make too much hormone.

⊙ Thyroiditis. A problem with the immune system or a viral infection[3] causes the thyroid gland to become inflamed and produce extra thyroid hormone that leaks into the bloodstream.

How Is Hyperthyroidism Treated?

There are several treatments for hyperthyroidism. Your doctor will choose an appropriate treatment based on your age, your physical condition, the cause of your hyperthyroidism and how severe your condition is.[4]

⊙ Radioactive iodine. Radioactive iodine is taken by mouth. It gets into the blood stream and is absorbed by overactive thyroid cells.

⊙ Anti-thyroid medicine. These drugs treat hyperthyroidism by blocking the thyroid's ability to produce hormones.

⊙ Surgery. Hyperthyroidism can be treated with a surgery (called a thyroidectomy) in which your doctor removes most of your thyroid gland.[5] After surgery, you will need to take a thyroid hormone supplement to restore your hormone levels to normal.

⊙ Beta blockers. No matter what other method of treatment you use, your physician may prescribe a beta blocker drug to slow your heart rate and reduce palpitations, shaking and nervousness until your thyroid levels are closer to normal.

Notes

1. Adam's apple

喉结。《圣经·创世纪》说，上帝创造了人类的祖先亚当（Adam）和夏娃（Eve）之后，让他们住在伊甸园（Eden）里，并且告诫他们：绝对不可以吃智慧之树的果实。结果，Eve 听信了魔鬼的唆使，不仅自己吃了禁果，还拿给 Adam 吃。正当他们大吃苹果的时候，上帝突然出现了，不由分说就把他们逐出了伊甸园。

其实古代西方人泛指所有的果实为 apple，而男性的喉结看起来比女性明显，人们以为这是因为 Adam 来不及咽下的苹果还留在喉咙里的缘故。所以，"Adam's apple" 就用来形容"男性的喉结"了。

2. Hyperthyroidism usually begins slowly, so its symptoms can be mistaken for stress or other health problems.

"be mistaken for" …被误认为…；短语 "mistake A for B" 的意思为"把 A 误认为 B"，亦可以用做 be mistaken for，即：A is mistaken for B.

Kindness is easily mistaken for love.

The traveler mistook the house for a hotel.

= The house was mistaken for a hotel.

3. 构成名词的部分常见后缀

名词后缀	– ness	– ity	– tion
n.	nervousness weakness	irritability sensitivity	perspiration
adj. /v.	nervous weak	irritable sensitive	perspire

4. Your doctor will choose an appropriate treatment based on your age，your physical condition，the cause of your hyperthyroidism and how severe your condition is.

"based on"之后带了四个并列成分，并列时保持并列部分的语法结构相同或相似。"how severe your condition is"为名词性从句，与之前三个名词保持了一致。

5. Hyperthyroidism can be treated with a surgery（called a thyroidectomy）in which your doctor removes most of your thyroid gland.

"in which…"为介词 + 关系词引导的定语从句。关键一：介词的选择。介词的判断可将先行词放入后面从句中，看用什么介词将其与句子连接起来，尤其是一些动词 + 介词的搭配。关键二：介词的位置。多数介词可以置于关系词前也可置于从句末，但短语动词的介词不可提前。如：He is the man who I am looking for. 该句中的介词 for 便不可提到关系词 who 之前。

Glossary

Word	English definition	Example
perspiration *n.*	drops of liquid that form on your skin when you are hot	Beads of perspiration stood out on his forehead
tremor *n.*	a slight shaking movement in a part of your body caused，for example，by cold or fear	There was a slight tremor in his voice
irritability *n.*	an irritable petulant（bad-tempered）feeling v. irritate adj. irritable	It was the almost furtive restlessness and irritability that had possessed him
fatigue *n.*	a feeling of being extremely tired，usually because of hard work or exercise	I was dropping with fatigue and could not keep my eyes open
pound *v.*	（of heart/blood）to beat quickly and loudly	Her heart was pounding with excitement
swell *v.*	（swelled，swollen）to become bigger or rounder	Her arm was beginning to swell up where the bee had stung her
subtle *adj.*	（often）not very noticeable or obvious	There are subtle differences between the two versions
bulge *v.*	to stick out from something in a round shape	His eyes bulged
blurry *adj.*	without a clear outline；not clear v. blur	My blurry vision makes it hard to drive
inflamed *adj.*	（of a part of the body）red，sore and hot because of infection or injury	Her joints are severely inflamed
radioactive *adj.*	sending out harmful radiation caused when the nuclei of atoms are broken up	The waste is safely locked away until it is no longer radioactive
menstrual *adj.*	connected with the time when a woman menstruates each month	This is the beginning of your first menstrual cycle

Word	English definition	Example
autoimmune *adj.*	a disease or medical condition is one which is caused by substances that usually prevent illness	I can prove an autoimmune disease in five minutes
immune *adj.*	not affected by a given influence	The immune system is our main defence against disease

Word	English definition	Chinese definition
hyperthyroidism *n.*	a condition in which the thyroid is overactive, making growth and mental development faster than normal	甲状腺功能亢进
thyroid *n.*	a small organ at the front of the neck that produces hormones that control the way in which the body grows and functions	甲状腺
gland *n.*	an organ in a person's or an animal's body that produces a substance for the body to use. There are many different glands in the body.	腺
hormone *n.*	a chemical substance produced in the body or in a plant that encourages growth or influences how the cells and tissues function	激素；荷尔蒙
metabolism *n.*	the chemical processes in living things that change food, etc. into energy and materials for growth	新陈代谢
bowel *n.*	the tube along which food passes after it has been through the stomach, especially the end where waste is collected before it is passed out of the body	肠
ophthalmopathy *n.*	an eye disease	眼病变
nodule *n.*	a small round lump or swelling, especially on a plant	结节；小瘤
lump *n.*	a swelling under the skin, sometimes a sign of serious illness	肿块，隆起
thyroiditis *n.*	inflammation of the thyroid gland	甲状腺炎
iodine *n.*	a nonmetallic element belonging to the halogens; used especially in medicine and photography and in dyes; occurs naturally only in combination in small quantities (as in sea water or rocks)	碘
palpitations *n.*	a physical conditionin which your heart beats very quickly and in an irregular way	心悸

Post – reading

A1. True/False/Not Given

Refer to the passage and look at the statements below. Write

YES　　　　　　if the statement agrees with the writer;

NO　　　　　　if the statement does not agree with the writer;

NOT GIVEN　　if there is no information about this in the passage.

1. The thyroid gland is located at the back of your neck.

2. Hyperthyroidism can be mistaken for stress or other health problems.

3. Hyperthyroidism definitely causes eye problems.

4. In more than half of cases, hyperthyroidism is caused by an autoimmune disorder called Graves' disease.

5. You can decide what kind of treatment will be done to your hyperthyroidism.

A2. Scan and complete the sentences.

1. Hyperthyroidism means your thyroid gland ＿＿＿＿＿ and ＿＿＿＿＿ too much thyroid hormone.

2. It is ＿＿＿＿＿ that control your metabolism.

3. Older adults may have subtle symptoms, such as ＿＿＿＿＿, ＿＿＿＿＿ and ＿＿＿＿＿ during normal activities.

4. An ＿＿＿＿＿ disease is when your immune system produces ＿＿＿＿＿ that attack your body's ＿＿＿＿＿ and/or organs.

5. Two other common causes of hyperthyroidism are ＿＿＿＿＿ and ＿＿＿＿＿ .

B1. Choose the appropriate word and fill in the blank with its correct form.

irritability	pound	subtle	inflame
fatigue	bulge	blurry	perspiration

1. Chronic ＿＿＿＿＿ is also one of the salient features of depression.

2. His heart was ＿＿＿＿＿, as if he were frightened.

3. His glasses magnified his ＿＿＿＿＿ glare.

4. During fever a large quantity of fluid is lost in ＿＿＿＿＿ .

5. The policeman's gun left an obvious ＿＿＿＿＿ under his coat.

6. The slow and ＿＿＿＿＿ changes take place in all living things.

7. Her question seemed to ＿＿＿＿＿ him all the more.

8. Something dark and ＿＿＿＿＿ came out and fixed its bug-eyes on me.

B2. Choose the proper explanation.

Word	Explanation
a. hormone	i. the failure of an organism in recognizing its own constituent parts as self, thus leading to an immune response against its own cells and tissues
b. thyroid gland	ii. an abnormality of heartbeat characterized by simultaneous awareness of one's pulse and discomfort
c. metabolism	iii. the set of life-sustaining chemical transformations within the cells of living organisms
d. autoimmune	iv. a class of regulatory biochemical that is produced by glands, and transported by the circulatory system to a distant target organ to coordinate its physiology and behavior
e. palpations	v. the gland that controls how quickly the body uses energy, makesproteins, and controls how sensitive the body is to other hormones

B3. Guess meaning from prefix and suffix.

hyper – 超过，太多 hypo – 下面，次等

hyperthyroidism – _____ hypertension – _____

hypothyroidism – _____ hypotension – _____

– itis 炎症

thyroiditis – _____ bronchitis – _____

meningitis – _____ tonsillitis – _____

C1. Multiple choice

1. Cathy is taking notes of the grammatical rules in class at Sunshine School, where she _____ English for a year.

    A. studies   B. studied

    C. is studying   D. has been studying

2. —I have got a headache.

    —No wonder. You _____ in front of that computer too long.

    A. work   B. are working

    C. have been working   D. worked

3. —Hi, Tracy, you look pale.

    —I am tired. I _____ the living room all day.

    A. painted   B. had painted

    C. have been painting   D. have painted

4. — I'm sure Andrew will win the first prize in the final.

    — I think so. He _____ for it for months.

    A. is preparing   B. was preparing

    C. had been preparing   D. has been preparing

5. The unemployment rate in this district _____ from 6% to 5% in the past two years.

    A. has fallen   B. had fallen

    C. is falling   D. was falling

C2. Fill in the blank with an appropriate preposition.

1. The book, _____ which he paid 6 Yuan, is worth reading.

2. The little girl is reading a book, _____ which there are many pictures.

3. Wu Dong, _____ whom I went to the concert, enjoyed it very much.

4. The speed _____ which you drive your car mustn'tbe too high.

5. The villagers dug along tunnel _____ which they could go to the fields without being found by the Japanese soldiers.

C3. Fill in the blanks with a preposition + relative pronoun.

1. The emperor, _____ the palace was built, was very cruel.

2. The money, _____ he bought the bike, was given by his grandfather.

3. The story, _____ the film is based, is a true one.

4. He spent a wonderful summer, _____ he joined us in the camping trip.

5. It is a family of 8 children, all _____ are studying music.

C4. Make sentences using relative clauses with preposition + relative pronoun.

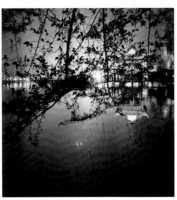

（West Lake is a beautiful place.
Hangzhou is famous for this place.）

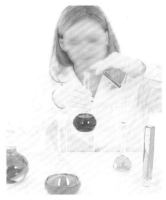

（The scientist went abroad last week.
My father worked with him）

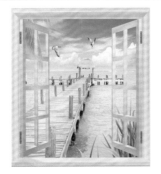

（There is a big window in my room.
I can see lovely sea through it.）

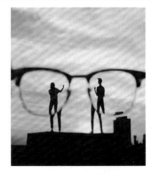

（I lost my glasses.
I could see nothing without them）

C5. Translation

1. 她经常被认为是她的双胞胎妹妹。（mistake）

2. 不同的细菌种类对抗菌素青霉素的反应很不同。（sensitivity）

3. 他们爱炫耀，几乎对每种情况都添油加醋。（tendency）

4. 人们会由于种种原因改变主意。（a variety of）

5. 该词典的补编或许将于明年出版。（supplement）

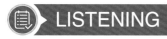 LISTENING

Part A　Listen carefully and finish the following sentences with "True" or "False". 听力

1. Stella, who is forty-four years old, comes from California.

2. To battle the disease, Stella visited many doctors over the world.

3. She expected that the US would be able to help her but she was frustrated that they cannot help her.

4. Stella found the Chinese doctor Xiao Haipeng through the net.

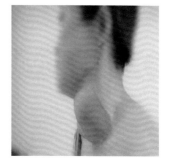

5. It has estimated that over forty people have been killed in Guangzhou with this method.

Part B　Complete the sentences within NO MORE THAN THREE WORDS.

1. She has suffered this disease for _____ .

2. The symptoms include _____ , _____ , palpitation and thyroid enlargement.

3. Due to her _____ to some medicines, Stella was told doctors cannot do anything to help her.

4. Xiao Haipeng thinks that _____ is very contraindicated. "

5. _____ is a dominated surgery in China for over 10 years.

6. It is a much safer procedure compared traditional surgery without _____ .

7. Stella is confident that more patients could _____ international exchange of medical expertise.

书网融合······

微课1

微课2

微课3

自测题

PPT

Unit 12 Acne

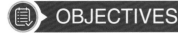

OBJECTIVES

When you have completed Unit 12, you will be able to

⊙ understand and identify professional terms related to acne.

⊙ communicate with the doctor about the treatment of acne.

⊙ get the main idea by skimming the passage.

⊙ describe the causes and treatments of acne.

⊙ tell your friends how to deal with the acne pain.

⊙ master the use of demonstrative pronoun.

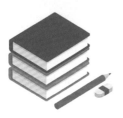

LEAD IN

Acne is a confusing skin disorder that affects tens of millions of people all over the world. Even with what we know about acne, many people still have questions they need answered.

Can you answer the following questions?

人家都说长痘千万不能去挤它

也一直幻想如果自己皮肤很好……

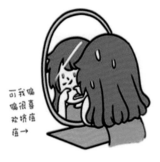

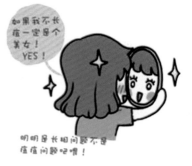

Q1: Is acne a cause of not cleaning yourself?

Q2: Are teenagers the only ones to get acne?

Q3: Is there really a way to prevent acne?

Q4: What can honestly be done about acne?

Q5: How long does it take acne to clear up?

CONVERSATION

会话

Betty: Good morning, doctor!

Doctor: Good morning!

Betty: I have a serious acne problem, doctor! I was a waitress and I was fired by my boss.

Doctor: Let me see. [After examining Betty] It doesn't seem very serious. I will prescribe a box of Doxycycline for you.

Betty: How long do I use this cream before I see results?

Doctor: All acne treatments take weeks to months to see results. Hang in there as you will be using treatment for a long time before you see positive results.

Betty: When will my acne go away?

Doctor: Acne is the worst during adolescence and will resolve as you head into adulthood. As I mentioned above adult acne can occur between ages 20 ~ 40.

Betty: I have blackheads, is that treated differently?

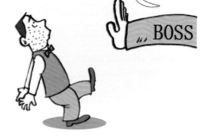

Acne affect gueata appetite,you are firod

BOSS

Doctor: Yes. For blackheads, we need a different treatment. Remember to touch your face as little as possible, so as not to add oils or put pressure on the skin. And avoid the urge to burst pimples. This can leave permanent marks on the skin. Also avoid strong soaps, and to be gentle as you wash and dry your skin.

Betty: I see. Thank you very much. I'll obey the rules and take care of myself!

Activity

Suppose your close friend has a serious acne problem. What should he/she pay attention to?

READING

Acne

Pre – reading

What is acne?

Where can acne develop?

Who getsacne?

What are the common acne causes?

How to treat acne?

While – reading

What Is Acne?

Acne is one of the most common skin disorders. The most common form of acne is called acne vulgaris.[1]

Acne is a disease of hair follicles and develops in stages. Beginning with blackheads and whiteheads acne may develop into large nodules and cysts. Acne not only disfigures skin, but also affects the psychology of the person suffering from it. That is why it is important to treat it as soon as possible.

In the first stage, acne begins as whiteheads and blackheads. Blackheads are called open comedones and whiteheads are called closed comedones.

The second stage of Acne is pimples or zits. They are also known as papules and pustules. Pimples form when the plugged pores get inflamed. When pimples get further infected and inflamed, the third stage of acne develops. These are called as nodules and cysts.

Acne will not always develop into the more severe stages. It may stop growing after the first stage.

Common Acne Causes

Heredity

If you have a family history of acne, you are at a greater risk of getting acne. Acne is not strictly hereditary, but the probability is higher if your family has a history of acne.

Hormones

Androgen group hormones activate the sebaceous glands and also help block pore openings. Hormonal changes during puberty therefore trigger acne. This is the main cause of acne in teenagers. Women may get acne at later ages because of changes in hormones.

Oily skin

Those with oily skin have a greater probability of getting acne.[2] The excess sebum may also block pore openings.

Food

Though no food is directly

linked with acne, experience

suggests that some people get acne from eating certain foods.[3] If you find any association between a food and your acne, stop eating that food.

Pressure and sweating

Pressure, rubbing of the skin and sweating can cause an acne

Menstrual cycle

Women may get acne some days before the beginning of their menstrual cycle because of changes in their hormones.

Medicines

Some medicines can cause acne break-out.

Cosmetics and skin care products

Acne can be caused by the use of cosmetics.

Where Can Acne Develop?

Acne can develop on all the places of the body where hair follicles are located. The density of follicles is greater on the face, neck, chest, back, shoulders, neck and upper arms. Acne is therefore most common on face, arms and trunk.

Who Gets Acne?

Mostly teenagers suffers from acne, but people of any age can get it. Acne can affect people in their thirties, forties or above.

Acne: Treatments

To treat acne, we have to address its causes:

⊙ the blocking of the follicle pore

⊙ presence of bacterium Pacnes inside the follicle and

⊙ excess sebum production.

The above changes occur because of hormonal imbalance, use of comedogenic products and other reasons.

Medicines are used to treat one or more of these causes. The choice of medication will depend upon the severity of acne and the possible reason of its formation. Hormonal treatment may be used for women who get acne due to hormonal imbalance. Antibiotics may be used if the acne is infected. Thus we use the medication depending upon the cause and condition of the outbreak.

Acne may be treated with –

⊙ topical creams, gels, liquids etc.

⊙ oral medicines such as antibiotics, Isotretinoin and Nicotinamide

⊙ physical and surgical procedures

⊙ light and laser therapy

Notes

1. The most common form of acne is called acne vulgaris.

vulgaris 是形容词，译为"寻常的"。文中短语 acne vulgaris 是寻常痤疮；普通粉刺的意思。

如：No, I will get acne vulgaris in my beautiful face.

不，吃那个我漂亮的脸蛋会长痘痘的。

2. Those with oily skin have a greater probability of getting acne.

这里的 those 指代的是 those people。

Those 能代替前面提到的同名异物中特指的事物，只能指代复数名词，相当于 the ones。如：

In China, students learn English at school as a foreign language, except for those in Hong Kong, where many people speak English as a first or a second language. （those 代替复数名词 students）

The computers in your office are more expensive than those / the ones in our school. （those 代替复数名词 computers）

3. Though no food is directly linked with acne, experience suggests that some people get acne from eating certain foods.

is linked with 译为"与…有联系的"

如：But over the last few years researchers have noticed that obesity in middle age is linked with cognitive problems in the aged.

然而在过去几年里研究人员发现中年肥胖与老年时发生认知障碍有关联．。

The UN is interested in partnerships where corporate capacity is linked with key areas of interest.

联合国对将公司能力与重要利益领域进行关联的合作感兴趣。

The dietary change was also shown to cause the kidneys to release more of a protein called renin and its hormone aldosterone which is linked with high blood pressure.

饮食的改变也使肾脏分泌出更多的蛋白质称为肾激素，它的激素醛固酮与高血压密切相关。

Glossary

Word	English definition	Example
disorder *n.*	condition in which there is a disturbance of normal functioning	Do the best that you can and be proud of yourself for having the courage to continue to fight your eating disorder
disfigure *v.*	mar or spoil the appearance	Every year, about 150 Africans are diagnosed with leprosy, a disease that disfigures the skin and affects the nervous system
blocked *adj.*	completely obstructed or closed off	Jane blocked Cross's vision and he could see nothing
inflamed *adj.*	resulting from inflammation; hot and swollen and reddened	So, while a good wash with soap and water is still a great idea, overwashing might lead to some unpleasant symptoms, not to mention inflamed and unsightly hands
density *n.*	the amount per unit size	The population density of that country is 685 per square mile
heredity *n.*	the biological process whereby genetic factors are transmitted from one generation to the next	Some diseases are present by heredity
vulgaris *adj.*	a Latin adjective meaning common, or something that is derived from the masses of common people	No, I will get acne vulgaris in my beautiful face
sebaceous *adj.*	containing an unusual amount of grease or oil	However, because of more active sebaceous glands, men's skin tends to be much oilier
menstrual *adj.*	of or relating to menstruation or the menses	This is the beginning of your first menstrual cycle

Word	English definition	Chinese definition
comedo *n.*	a black-tipped plug clogging a pore of the skin	粉刺；面疱 复数 comedones
androgen *n.*	male sex hormone that is produced in the testes and responsible for typical male sexual characteristics	雄性激素；男性荷尔蒙
pacnes *n.*	corynebaterium acnes	痤疮丙酸杆菌 propionibacterium acnes 缩写
comedogenic *adj.*	prone to blackheads	易生黑头粉刺的
isotretinoin *n.*	a drug related to vitamin A, used to treat severe acne that has failed to respond to other treatment	（用来治疗严重痤疮的） 异维 A 酸
nicotinamide *n.*	nicotinic acid amide	烟酰胺；烟碱
hormone *n.*	the secretion of an endocrine gland that is transmitted by the blood to the tissue on which it has a specific effect	激素；荷尔蒙 复数 hormones

Word	English definition	Chinese definition
pimple *n.*	a small inflamed elevation of the skin; a pustule or papule; common symptom in acne	丘疹，面疱 复数 pimples
zit *n.*	a small inflamed elevation of the skin; a pustule or papule; common symptom in acne	青春痘；粉刺 复数 zits
hair follicles *n.*	one appendix organ of skin, play an important role in skin self-renewing hair growth and tumor origin	毛囊
psychology *n.*	the science of mental life	心理学；心理状态 复数 psychologies
sebum *n.*	the oily secretion of the sebaceous glands; with perspiration it moistens and protects the skin	皮脂
bacterium *n.*	single-celled or noncellular spherical or spiral or rod-shaped organisms lacking chlorophyll that reproduce by fission	细菌 复数 bacteria
antibiotics *n.*	a chemical substance derivable from a mold or bacterium that kills microorganisms and cures infections	抗生素

Post – reading

A1. Scan the text and complete the sentence.

1. Acne is a disease of hair follicles and develops in ＿＿＿＿＿＿ .

2. Acne not only ＿＿＿＿＿＿ skin, but also ＿＿＿＿＿＿ the psychology of the person suffering from it.

3. If you have a family history of acne, you are at a greater risk of ＿＿＿＿＿＿

＿＿＿＿＿＿ .

4. Women may get acne at later ages because of changes in ＿＿＿＿＿＿ .

5. Women may get acne some days before the beginning of their ＿＿＿＿＿＿

＿＿＿＿＿＿ because of changes in their hormones.

6. The choice of medication will depend upon the ＿＿＿＿＿＿ acne and the possible reason of its formation.

A2. Decide whether the following sentences are true or false.

1. Only teenagers suffer from acne, people in their thirties, forties or above won't get it.

2. Acne not only disfigures skin, but also affects the psychology of the person.

3. The risk of getting acne has nothing to do with a family history.

4. Women may get acne at later ages because of changes in hormones.

5. When choosing medication, we should understand the severity of acne and the possible

reason of its formation.

B1. Match the following words with their English meaning.

Word	Meaning
1. pore	a. put in motion or move to act
2. activate	b. any tiny hole admitting passage of a liquid (fluid or gas)
3. follicle	c. a quantity much larger than is needed
4. sebum	d. any small spherical group of cells containing a cavity
5. cyst	e. the oily secretion of the sebaceous glands; with perspiration it moistens and protects the skin
6. excess	f. a closed sac that develops abnormally in some body structure

B2. Fill in the blanks with the words in the text. The first letter is given to you.

1. If you have an underlying d _____ go to the doctor.

2. Therefore, it is wise to keep away from anger or shun anger. Anger instigates bitterness, shatters friendship, d _____ our composure, converts wisdom into folly and destroys fame and glory.

3. If you have tried all of the routes above and are still b _____ and frustrated then find a job elsewhere.

4. The increasing population d _____ will even further congeal traffic.

5. For some it becomes a family h _____ and for some a single son or daughter gain popularity even though in the family there are some handicaps.

B3. Guess meaning from prefix and make some examples.

disorder   disease   disfigure   dis – _____

1. dis _____ _____   2. dis _____ _____

3. dis _____ _____   4. dis _____ _____

5. dis _____ _____   6. dis _____ _____

C1. Choose the best answer for the following exercise.

1. The New English-Chinese Dictionary has been republished several times, _____ edition more up to date than the last.

    A. any   B. everyone   C. either   D. each

2. After paying $1,000 _____, you'll all become full members of our club.

    A. each   B. all   C. every   D. both

3. _____ was her cruelty that we all hated about her.

    A. It   B. What   C. That   D. Such

4. Mary has been ill in bed for a week. I wonder if she is _____ better now.

    A. much   B. some   C. any   D. very

5. – Which of these two ties will you take?　　– I don't like these. Do you have any _____?

A. one   B. other   C. ones   D. others

6. I'd rather ride a bike as bike riding has _____ of the trouble of taking buses.

    A. much   B. all   C. neither   D. none

7. I need some blue ink today but there is _____ at hand.

    A. not   B. nothing   C. a little   D. none

8. I found my watch _____ I had left _____ .

    A. where, it   B. that, it   C. which, one   D. where, one

9. I don't have time to get the tickets. Who's going to _____ ?

    A. do so   B. do it   C. buy it   D. do them

10.   – Jack certainly has a high opinion of Susan. It can't be better than _____ of him.

    A. hers   B. she   C. that   D. her

C2. Write the antonym of the following words by adding the proper prefixes.

1. agreeable	11. human
2. content	12. correct
3. courage	13. justice
4. legal	14. sincere
5. logical	15. accurate
6. legible	16. lucky
7. mortal	17. conditional
8. moral	18. limited
9. regular	19. tie
10. rational	20. pack

C3. Translate the following sentences into English.

1. 让我们分配粮食给最需要的人。

2. 你的工资可以按周以现金支取，或按月以支票支取。二者可选其一。

3. 这个仪式对于那些新近丧失亲友的人来说是一种折磨。

4. 手工制品受到那些已厌倦划一产品的人的欢迎。

5. 只有 70 岁以上的人才有资格领取这项专款。

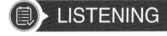 **LISTENING**

听力

Fill in the blanks according to what you hear.

1. A popular treatment for acne is the _____ _____ _____

_____, which calms down the inflammation. Also, the hole that's made during the injection can also _____ _____ _____ _____ _____

because some of the puss and the keratin plug that is causing the acne and inflammation can

_____ _____ . Sometimes a larger needle is used to drain the lesion, because

that's the primary way you're going to treat the _____ _____ .

2. If you're at home and you can't get to a doctor, some things that you can do to help

with these deep, painful lesions are: 1) if it's early, the lesion is about to form, you can

_____ _____ to the area for a few minutes to _____ _____

the inflammation, much like mostly teenagers would do if you _____ _____

_____ doing a sport.

3. If the lesion is _____ and it looks like it's starting to come to a head and it's

more _____ , apply heat may help, like you might do with a boil, to get it to come to

a head and _____ .

4. Sometimes taking _____ at home, if that's something that you're able to do and

that's safe for you, can help with some of the _____ of an acne lesion.

书网融合……

微课 1	微课 2	微课 3	自测题

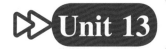 **Unit 13** **Vitamin Deficiency**

PPT

Objectives

When you have completed Unit 13, you will be able to

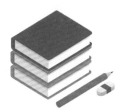

⊙ Understand and identify professional terms related to vitamin deficiency.

⊙ Communicate with the chemist about the use of vitamins.

⊙ Understand the meaning of the common affixes

⊙ skim the passage for main idea.

⊙ Describe symptoms, causes and treatment of folate deficiency.

⊙ obtain main points by listening to the lecture.

⊙ master the use of restrictive attributive clause.

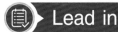 Lead in

Vitamins are needed for the proper functioning of our body. They help in keeping our eyes, bones, teeth, and gums healthy. There are 13 vitamins, each of which has a specific function.

Lack of vitamins in the body can cause deficiency diseases. It is also called vitamin deficiency. Vitamin deficiency is a group of diseases caused by the deficiency of one or more vitamins. Symptoms depend on the type and degree of vitamin deficiency.

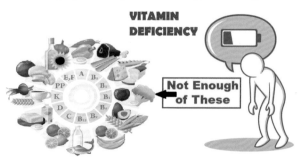

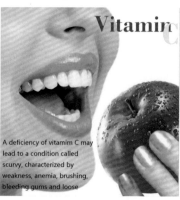

Can you answer the following questions?

Q1：What are the main functions of vitamin

Q2：What can be caused by lacking of vitamins in the body?

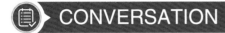 **CONVERSATION**

会话

Betty enters a drugstore on a Sunday morning.

Pharmacist：Good morning, can I help you?

Betty：Good morning! I want to buy vitamins of some kind. It is said that vitamins are good for health.

Pharmacist：What kind of vitamin do you want?

Betty：I'm not very sure. Can you introduce some to me?

Pharmacist：Sure. Vitamin A prevents eye problems, promotes a healthy immune system, is

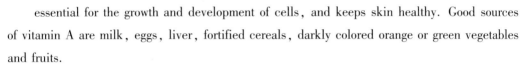

essential for the growth and development of cells, and keeps skin healthy. Good sources of vitamin A are milk, eggs, liver, fortified cereals, darkly colored orange or green vegetables and fruits.

Betty：Thanks. What about vitamin C?

Pharmacist：Vitamin C is needed to form collagen, a tissue that helps to hold cells together. It's essential for healthy bones, teeth, gums, and blood vessels. It helps the body absorb iron, aids in wound healing, and contributes to brain function. You'll find high levels of vitamin C in citrus fruits, strawberries, kiwi, guava, peppers, tomatoes, broccoli, and spinach.

Betty：Thank you very much. And they say taking vitamin E can make one young.

Pharmacist：Yes. Vitamin E is an antioxidant and helps protect cells from damage. It is also important for the health of red blood cells. Vitamin E is found in many foods, such as vegetable oils, nuts, and green leafy vegetables. Avocados, wheat germ, and whole grains are also good sources.

Betty：I see. So I can get enough vitamins from the daily food?

Pharmacist：Yes, there is no need to take extra vitamins every day.

Betty：Thank you very much.

Pharmacist：You are welcome.

Activity

Practice the dialogue, discuss the function ofvitamin A, vitamin C, vitamin E and say something about vitamin D.

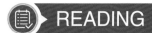
READING

Pre – reading

What is folate deficiency?

What are the symptoms of folate deficiency?

How can folate deficiency be treated?

While – reading

What is folate (vitamin B_9) deficiency?

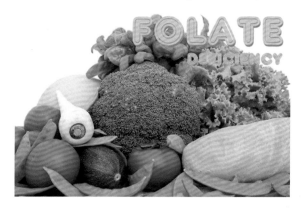

Vitamin B_9, also called folate or folic acid, is a type of B vitamin.

Folate is the naturally occurring form of vitamin B_9. Folic acid is the synthetic version of vitamin B_9, which is found in fortified foods and supplements.

Vitamin B_9 plays an essential role in:

· making and repairing your DNA

· producing red blood cells

If you don't have enough folate in your diet, you may end up with a folate deficiency. Folate deficiency is common, and associated with numerous health problems.

Symptoms of folate deficiency

The symptoms offolate deficiency include:

· tiredness

· weakness

· heart palpitations

· shortness of breath

· headaches

· irritability

· difficulty concentrating

If you have any of these symptoms, it's really important to test your levels.

Effects offolate deficiency

Folate deficiency Anaemia

You need folate to make normal red blood cells, so if you're deficient it can lead to megaloblastic anaemia — where your red blood cells are not fully developed and larger than usual. This means you can't transport enough oxygen around your body.

Neural tube defects

Folate plays an essential role in the development of a baby's brain and spinal cord during pregnancy. If you're deficient, especially in the first few weeks of pregnancy, it might lead to a serious birth defect called a neural tube defect (NTD).

If you have low levels of folate during pregnancy, it might increase your risk of premature labour or your baby could have a low birth weight.

Heart disease

Folate plays an important role in homocysteine metabolism. If you don't have enough folate to help metabolise and lower your homocysteine levels, it might increase your risk for heart disease.

Causes offolate deficiency

Your body can't build up a store offolate so you can become deficient in a matter of weeks. So it's important to continuously get enough from your diet or from supplements.

You might also be at an increased risk of folate deficiency if you:

· are pregnant

· have a poor diet

· drink excessive amounts of alcohol

· take certain medications — like anticonvulsants and proton pump inhibitors (PPIs)

· have a gastrointestinal disorder — like coeliac or Crohn's disease

· have a genetic disorder that stops your body from convertingfolate to a form your body can use

How to treat folate deficiency

Folate (vitamin B$_9$) deficiency can be treated by increasing the amount of folate – rich foods you eat or by taking a folic acid supplement.

Folate – rich foods

Even if you're thinking of taking a folic acid supplement, including folate – rich foods in your diet is a good idea. These foods are full of other nutrients and are good for your overall health. Foods high in folate include：

· leafy, green vegetables — for example, spinach, kale, broccoli, cabbage, and Brussels sprouts

· beans, peas, and lentils

· eggs

· shellfish

· beetroot

· oranges

· wholegrains

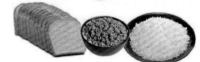

Foods High in Folate

Fortified bread, cereals and rice

Beans   Orange juice   Spinach

Foods fortified with folic acid

Some foods, particularly some breakfast cereals, are fortified with folic acid. You'll be able to see this on the food label.

Folic acid supplements

For most people, taking a folic acid supplement for about four months is enough. You might need to continue taking them if your levels still aren't back to normal after this.

Notes

1. deficiency   n. 缺乏

de 是前缀，表示不，非，使相反，是一种派生法。所谓派生法，就是在词根前加前缀或在其后加后缀构成新词。加前缀，一般不改变词性，而只是引起词义上的变化。加后缀一般词义变化不大，只改变了词性。

其他常见前缀有 anti –（反对，相反，防止），auto –（自动，自己），co –（联合，伴同），bio –（生命，生物），extra –（以外，超过），fore –（前，先，预告），inter –（在......之间，互相），over –（过度），post –（后），pre –（前，预先），re –（回，再，重新），sub –（下，低于，次于），super –（超级，在......上，过度），tele –（远，电视），trans –（横过，转变，变换），vice –（副）。如：antioxidation 抗氧化剂，autodial 自动拨号，autocontrol 自动控制，biography 传记，coauthor 合著

者，coworker 同事，extraordinary 非凡的，extrabright 特别光亮的，forearm 前臂，foretell 预言，international 国际的，overstudy 用功过度，postflight 飞行后的，postwar 战后的，prehistory 史前，prewar 战前的，reconsider 重新考虑，repay 偿还，subway 地铁，super-bright 超亮的，supercool 过度冷却，superhero 超级英雄，telecontrol 遥控，telegraph 电报，transnational 超国界的，vice – chairman 副主席，vice – president 副总统。

2. You have a genetic disorder that stops your body from converting folate to a form your body can use.

此句是限定性定语从句，that 是关系代词。定语从句是由关系代词和关系副词引导的从句，其作用是作定语修饰主句的某个成分，定语从句分为限定性和非限定性从句两种。

在复合句中，修饰某一名词或代词，用作定语的从句叫做定语从句（attributive clause）。被定语从句所修饰的词叫做先行词（antecedent）。定语从句必须放在先行词之后。引导定语从句的关联词有关系代词 who、whom、whose、which、that 和关系副词 when、where、why 等。

Finally，the thief handed everything that he had stolen to the police. 最后，那个小偷向警察交出他偷的所有的东西。（引导词是关系代词 that）

His parents wouldn't let him marry anyone whose family was poor. 他父母不让他和家庭困难的人结婚。（引导词是关系代词 whose）

In the dark street，there wasn't a single person to whom she could turn for help. 在那个黑暗的街道上，没有她可以求助的人。（引导词是关系代词 whom）

In 1519 another traveller who went to America from Europe discovered the tomato. 1519 年另一位从欧洲去美洲的旅行家发现了西红柿。（引导词是关系代词 who）

I still remember the day when I first came to Beijing. 我仍然记得第一次去北京的那一天。（引导词是关系副词 when）

This is the house where we lived last year. 这就是我们去年住的房子。（引导词是关系副词 where）

Glossary

Word	English definition	Example
vitamin *n*.	any of a group of organic substances essential in small quantities to normal growth and nutrition.	Oranges are rich in vitamin C.
deficiency n.	a lack or insufficiency; shortage	They did blood tests on him for signs of vitamin deficiency.
tissue *n*.	part of an organism consisting of an aggregate of cells having a similar structure and function	As we age we lose muscle tissue.
vessel *n*.	an object used as a container (especially for liquids); a tube in which a body fluid circulates	The doctor burst a blood vessel.

续表

Word	English definition	Example
antioxidant *n.*	a substance which slows down the damage that can be caused to other substances by the effects of oxygen	Dates, cranberries and red grapes have high concentrations of antioxidants
normal *adj.*	conforming to a type, standard, or regular pattern	We are open during normal office hours.
concentrate *v.*	direct one's attention on something	She has been concentrating on her career.
fortified *adj.*	having something added to increase the strength	The explosion caused superficial damage to the fortified house.
supplement *n.*	a supplementary component that improves capability	It may also interact with some medications or supplements.

Word	English definition	Chinese definition
anaemia n.	a deficiency of red blood cells	贫血；贫血症
palpitation n.	a rapid and irregular heart beat	心悸；跳动；颤动
irritability n.	a disposition to exhibit uncontrolled anger	易怒；兴奋性
megaloblast n.	an abnormally large red blood cell precursor, present in certain types of anaemia	［临床］巨幼红细胞
spinal adj.	relating to your spine	脊髓的；脊柱的；
homocysteine n.	an amino acid occurring as an intermediate in the metabolism of methionine	半胱氨酸
metabolism n.	the way that chemical processes in your body cause food to be used in an efficient way, for example to make new cells and to give you energy	［生理］新陈代谢
anticonvulsant *n.*	a drug used to treat or prevent convulsions (as in epilepsy)	抗痉挛的，抗惊厥的
gastrointestinal adj.	relating to the stomach and the intestines.	胃肠的
crohn's disease *n.*	inflammation, thickening, and ulceration of any of various parts of the intestine	克罗恩病
citrus *n.*	any of numerous fruits of the genuscitrus having thick rind and juicy pulp	柑橘
kiwi *n.*	fuzzy brown egg‑shaped fruit with slightly tart green flesh	［植］猕猴桃；奇异果
broccoli *n.*	plant with dense clusters of tight green flower buds, plant with dense clusters of tight green flower buds	西兰花；花椰菜
spinach *n.*	dark green leaves, eaten cooked or raw in salads	菠菜

Post‑reading

A1. Scan the text and complete the sentence.

1. Vitamin B_9, also called folate or _____, is a type of B vitamin.

2. Vitamin B_9 plays an essential role in producing _____ _____ cells.

3. You might also be at an increased risk of folate deficiency if you drink excessive a-mounts of _____ .

4. Folate (Vitamin B_9) deficiency can be treated by _____ the amount of folate.

5. For most people, taking a folic acid supplement for about _____ months is e-nough.

6. You might need to continue taking them if your levels still aren't back to _____ after taking a folic acid supplement.

A2. Read the passage and answer the following questions.

1. What are the main functions of Vitamin B_9?

2. List at least three symptoms of folate deficiency.

3. What are the main effects of folate deficiency?

4. What kinds of vegetables contain high sources of Vitamin B_9?

5. How to treat folate deficiency?

B1. Match the following words with their English meaning.

Word	Meaning
1. vitamin	a. the organic processes (in a cell or organism) that are necessary for life
2. tissue	b. a disposition to exhibit uncontrolled anger
3. vessel	c. any of a group of organic substances essential in small quantities to normal growth and nutrition.
4. palpitation	d. part of an organism consisting of an aggregate of cells having a similar structure and function
5. metabolism	e. a tube in which a body fluid circulates
6. irritability	f. a rapid and irregular heart beat

B2. Fill in the blanks with the words in the text. The first letter is given to you.

1. If you don't have enough folate in your diet, you may end up with a folate d _____ .

2. The symptoms of folate deficiency include difficulty c _____ .

3. You need folate to make normal red blood cells, so if you're deficient it can lead to megaloblastic a _____ .

4. Folate plays an essential role in the development of a baby's brain and s _____ cord during pregnancy.

5. Even if you're thinking of taking a folic acid s _____ , including folate-rich foods in your diet is a good idea.

6. Some foods, particularly some breakfast cereals, are f _____ with folic acid.

B3. Guess meaning from prefixes and words.

pre- _____   fore- _____   inter- _____

preselect _____   forehead _____   interaction _____

sub-_____   over-_____   de-_____.

subway _____   overtime _____   degrade _____.

B4. Write the Chinese meaning of the following prefixes.

1. ab	6. co
2. anti	7. counter
3. auto	8. re
4. tele	9. extra
5. bio	10. super

C1. Choose the best answer for the following exercises.

1. Don't talk about such things of _____ you are not sure.

    A. which   B. what   C. as   D. those

2. Is this the factory _____ you visited the other day?

    A. that   B. where   C. in which   D. the one

3. Is this factory _____ some foreign friends visited last Friday?

    A. that   B. where   C. which   D. the one

4. Is this the factory _____ he worked ten years ago?

    A. that   B. where   C. which   D. the one

5. The wolves hid themselves in the places _____ couldn't be found.

    A. that   B. where   C. in which   D. in that

6. The freezing point is the temperature _____ water changes into ice.

    A. at which   B. on that   C. in which   D. of what

7. This book will show you _____ can be used in other contexts.

    A. how you have observed

    B. what you have observed

    C. that you have observed

    D. how that you have observed

8. The reason is _____ he is unable to operate the machine.

    A. because   B. why   C. that   D. whether

9. I'll tell you _____ he told me last week.

    A. all which   B. that   C. all that   D. which

10. That tree, _____ branches are almost bare, is very old.

    A. whose   B. of which   C. in which   D. on which

11. I have bought the same dress _____ she is wearing.

    A. as   B. that   C. which   D. what

12. He failed in the examination, _____ made his father very angry.

A. which　　　　B. it　　　　C. that　　　　D. what

13. We're talking about the piano and the pianist _____ were in the concert we attended last night.

A. which　　　B. whom　　　C. who　　　D. that

14. The girl _____ an English song in the next room is Tom's sister.

A. who is singing　B. is singing　　C. sang　　　D. was singing

15. Those _____ not only from books but also through practice will succeed.

　A. learn　　B. who　　　C. that learns　　D. who learn

C2.　Translation

1. 叶酸可溶于水。

2. 它还添加了维生素 B_9。

3. 我想要一间窗户朝海的房间。

4. 没有人知道他上学迟到的原因。

5. 叶酸补充过量可能危害你的健康。

LISTENING

听力

Part A　Listen and answer the questions.

1. How many kinds of vitamins have scientists found?

2. If we do not get enough of the vitamins we need in our food, what kind of risk we will have?

3. What is Vitamin C needed for?

4. How many people are involved in the study on taking vitamin supplements?

5. What's your opinion on taking vitamin supplements every day?

Part B　Fill in the blanks according to what you hear. Write ONE WORD for each answer.

1. Much of our good health depends on the cooperation between _____. When they work together, chemical _____ take place smoothly. Body systems are kept in balance.

2. The word "vitamin" dates back to Polish scientist Casimir Funk in _____. He was studying a substance in the hull that covers _____. This substance was believed to cure a disorder called beriberi.

3. It is better to eat vitamin-rich foods to _____ disease instead of eating them to _____ a disease after it has developed.

4. People who do not get enough vitamin A can not see well in darkness. They may develop a condition that dries the eyes. This can result in _____ and lead to _____.

5. Vitamin B – one is also called thiamine. Thiamine changes starchy foods into energy.

It also helps the heart and _____ system work smoothly. Without it, we would be _____ and would not grow. We also might develop beriberi.

6. Vitamin D increases levels of the element calcium in the _____ . Calcium is needed for nerve and muscle cells to work _____ . It also is needed to build strong bones.

书网融合……

微课1   微课2   微课3   自测题

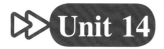 **Unit 14** **AIDS**

PPT

OBJECTIVES

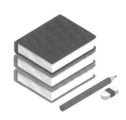

When you have completed Unit 14, you will be able to

⊙ understand and identify professional terms related to AIDS.

⊙ communicate with the doctor about some typical symptoms properly.

⊙ skim the passage for main idea.

⊙ describe the symptoms, the causes and the control of AIDS.

⊙ obtain information about AIDS by listening to the lecture.

⊙ master the structure "*It's up to sb to do sth*".

LEAD IN

What does the red ribbon symbolize?

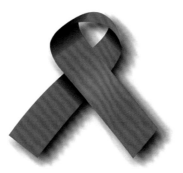

Can AIDS or HIV be transmitted by the following ways? Give your reason.

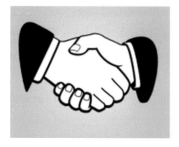

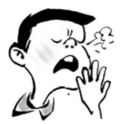

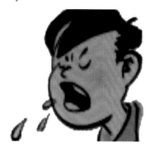

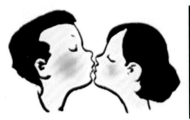
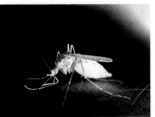
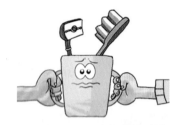

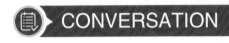

会话

Judy is an easygoing and warmhearted girl. She likes smiling and making friends. Two months ago, she was invited by her friend to take part in a special party which was organized by some HIV-positive patients. She knew that HIV or AIDS would not be transmitted by eating together. She went to the party. One month later, she felt uncomfortable. She caught a cold and red rash appeared on her skin. She began to worry and went to the hospital.

Doctor: Good morning, what's troubling you?

Judy: Good morning, doctor. I have felt terrible lately.

Doctor: What's wrong with you? Tell me more.

Judy: Er, I've been feeling rather uncomfortable. I have had so many colds and sore throats. My skin has broken out in an itchy rash. I am really worried about myself.

Doctor: OK, take it easy. Let me look at your red rash. How long have you had such symptom?

Judy: Er, about one month. At the beginning, there were only some spots on my arm, but now, the rash even spread to my neck and upper part of my breasts.

Doctor: Oh, it's so terrible. Do you feel itchy?

Judy: Sometimes, it is sore and itchy. But that's not the problem that I am really worrying about. The thing that I want to make it clear is whether I am infected with HIV virus or not.

Doctor: Why do you think so? Do you have some other symptoms?

Judy: Not yet. But I feel really bad these days. I thought maybe I am infected with HIV virus for I attended a party with some AIDS patients two months ago. We ate and drank together and even hugged each other after the party.

Doctor: It is impossible for you to be infected if you only ate and drank with them. There are many misconceptions about the transmission of AIDS or HIV, such as shaking hands, casual kissing, using the same toilet, eating together, and so on. Don't worry!

Judy: Oh, thank Goodness! I have been suffering a lot! But, doctor, why do I have so many spots on my skin.

Doctor: That's what I wanted to ask. Did you eat something unusual?

Judy：Nothing unusual, except some seafood.

Doctor：OK, maybe you are allergic to seafood or maybe it's just because of the toxins in the polluted air these days. I will prescribe you some ointment which is effective in treating skin rashes and allergies.

Judy：Thank you, doctor.

Doctor：You are welcome, bye!

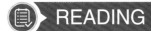 READING

AIDS

Pre – reading

What is the difference between HIV and AIDS?

What are the symptoms of early HIV infection?

What can we do to protect ourselves from AIDS?

While – reading

What Is AIDS?

AIDS (Acquired immune deficiency syndrome[1] or acquired immunodeficiency syndrome[2]) is a disease caused by a virus called HIV (Human Immunodeficiency Virus[3]). The illness alters the immune system[4], making people much more vulnerable to infections and diseases.

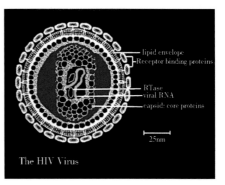

The HIV Virus

HIV is spread through contact with infected blood or fluids such as sexual secretions. Over time, the virus attacks the immune system, focusing on special cells called "CD_4 cells" which are important in protecting the body from infections and cancers, and the number of these cells starts to fall.[5] Eventually, the CD_4 cells fall to a critical level and/or the immune system is weakened so much that it can no longer fight off certain types of infections and cancers.

Both the virus and the disease are often referred to together as HIV/AIDS. People with HIV have what is called HIV infection. As a result, some will then develop AIDS. The development of numerous opportunistic infections in an AIDS patient can ultimately lead to death.

Symptoms

Many people with HIV have no symptoms for several years. Others may develop symptoms similar to flu, usually two to six weeks after catching the virus. Symptoms of early HIV infection may include:

⊙ fever

⊙ chills

⊙ joint pain

⊙ muscle ache

⊙ sore throat

⊙ sweats (particularly at night)

⊙ enlarged glands

⊙ a red rash

⊙ tiredness

⊙ weakness

⊙ weight loss

Transmission

HIV can be mainly transmitted through the following three channels:

⊙ sexual transmission. This can happen while having unprotected sex.

⊙ perinatal transmission.[6] The mother can pass the infection on to her child during childbirth, pregnancy, and also through breast feeding.

⊙ blood transmission. The risk of transmitting HIV through blood transfusion is nowadays extremely low.

⊙ individuals who give and receive tattoos and piercings are also at risk and should be very careful.

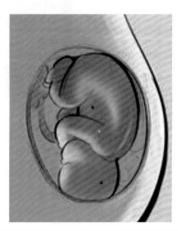

HIV vs AIDS

HIV is the virus which attacks the T-cells in the immune system.

AIDS is the syndrome which appears in advanced stages of HIV infection.

HIV is a virus.

AIDS is a medical condition.

HIV infection causes AIDS to develop. However, it is possible to be infected with HIV without developing AIDS. Without treatment, the HIV infection is allowed to progress and eventually it will develop into AIDS in the vast majority of cases.

Diagnosis

In 1985, a blood test became available that measures antibodies to HIV that are the body's immune system response to the HIV. This blood test remains the best method for diagnosing HIV infection. Recently, tests have become available to look for these same antibodies in blood and saliva, some providing results within 20 minutes of testing.[7]

A person can be infected with HIV without knowing it. So doctors recommend that anyone who thinks he or she may have been exposed to the virus get tested-even if the chance of having been infected seems small. Doctors test a person's blood to find out if he or she is infected with HIV.

Treatment

Right now there is no cure for HIV or AIDS. Scientists are also researching vaccines that may one day help to prevent HIV infection, but it is a very tough assignment, and no one knows when these vaccines might become available. It's up to everyone to prevent AIDS by avoiding the behaviors that lead to HIV infection.[8]

Notes

1. acquired immune deficiency syndrome 获得性免疫缺损综合征，艾滋病

2. acquired immunodeficiency syndrome 获得性免疫缺陷综合征

3. Human Immunodeficiency Virus 人类免疫缺陷病毒，艾滋病病毒

4. immune system 免疫系统

5. Over time, the virus attacks the immune system, focusing on special cells called "CD_4 cells" which are important in protecting the body from infections and cancers, and the number of these cells starts to fall.

这是一个并列复合句。第一句的主语是"the virus"，谓语是"attack"，宾语是"immune system"。"focusing on"现在分词短语在这里做方式状语，意为"专攻于"，此句中

还包含一个定语从句"which are important…cancers"用来修饰 CD$_4$ cells，"protected from…"指"保护…不受侵害或者伤害"例如，Wild wood should be well protect from excessive hag. 第二句话的主语是"the number of these cells"，主语中的 these cells 指代的是前一句中的 CD4 cells。这句话的谓语是"start to"。宾语是"fall"。

6. perinatal transmission 围产期传播

7. Recently，tests have become available to look for these same antibodies in blood and saliva，some providing results within 20 minutes of testing.

此句中副词"recently"表示"最近，近来"之意，强调时间点，多用过去时，例如，The bank recently opened a branch in German。表示时间长度，多用完成时，如，It is only fairly recently that historians have begun to investigate the question，需要注意的是 recently 不可用于将来时态中．"available"一词为"可用的，可获得的"英英释义为"If something you want or need is available，you can find it or obtain it．"例如，Cheap goods are available，but not in sufficient quantities to satisfy demand.

8. It's up to everyone to prevent AIDS by avoiding the behaviors that lead to HIV infection.

"It's up to sb to do sth"是 it 作形式主语的句型，一般有两种意思：①由某人决定去做某事，如：It's up to you to decide how to get there. ②做某事是某人的义务/职责/责任，如：It's up to her to lock the door. 本句中表示的是第二个意思，其中 it 是形式主语，不定式短语"to prevent AIDS by avoiding the behaviors that lead to HIV infection"是真正的主语"is up to everyone"是系表结构，做句子的谓语。不定式中，that lead to HIV infection 作定语来修饰 behavior. 整句话的意思是，每个人都有责任通过避免进行容易染上 HIV 病毒的行为来阻止艾滋病。

Glossary

Word	English definition	Example
ribbon *n.*	any long object resembling a thin line	This ribbon does not match with my hat
symbolize *v.*	express indirectly by an image，form，or model；be a symbol	Blue can symbolize trust and dependability
positive*adj.*	indicating existence or presence of a suspected condition or pathogen	All gram-positive bacteria are bounded by a single-unit lipid membrane
misconception *n.*	an incorrect conception	What is the most common misconception about your work
causal *adj.*	occurring or appearing by chance	We are the casual acquaintance of a long railway journey
alter *v.*	cause to change；make different	He is unlikely to alter his game plan
vulnerable *adj.*	be more likely to get a disease than other people，animals，or plants	People with high blood pressure are especially vulnerable to diabetes

Word	English definition	Example
Infect *v.*	to give someone a disease	People with the virus may feel perfectly well，but they can still infect others
critical *adj.*	situation that is very serious and dangerous	He remained in a critical condition after suffering heart failure
opportunistic *adj.*	taking immediate advantage，often unethically，of any circumstance of possible benefit	Cryptococcus infection is a common opportunistic infection in persons infected with human immunodeficiency virus（HIV）
transmit *v.*	transfer to another	Insects can transmit diseases
tattoo *n.*	a design that is drawn on someone's skin using needles to make little holes and filling them with colored dye	He has a tattoo on the back of his hand
expose *v.*	to put something in a situation where they are not protected from something dangerous or unpleasant	The report revealed that workers had been exposed to high levels of radiation
assignment *n.*	a duty that you are assigned to perform	He has just come off a difficult assignment

Word	English definition	Chinese definition
itchy adj.	causing an irritating cutaneous sensation；being affect with an itch	发痒的
syndrome *n.*	a pattern of symptoms indicative of some disease	综合征
infection *n.*	A disease caused by germs or bacteria	传染；感染；传染病
secretion *n.*	Liquid substances produced by parts of plants or bodies	分泌物
gland *n.*	Organ in the body which produces chemical substances for the body to use or get rid of	腺
rash *n.*	A lot of red spots on someone's skin，caused by an illness	皮疹
pregnancy *n.*	The condition of being pregnant or the period of time during which a female is pregnant.	怀孕；妊娠
blood transfusion *n.*	A process in which blood is injected into the body of a person who is badly injured or ill.	输血
diagnosis *n.*	The discovery and naming of what is wrong with someone who is ill or with something that is not working properly	诊断
antibody *n.*	Substances which a person's or an animal's body produces in their blood in order to destroy substances which carry disease	抗体
saliva *n.*	The watery liquid that forms in your mouth and helps you to chew and digest food.	唾液
vaccine *n.*	A substance containing a harmless form of the germs that cause a particular disease.	疫苗

Post – reading

A1. YES/NO/Not Given Questions

Refer to the passage and look at the statements below. Write

YES　　　　　　if the statement agrees with the writer；

NO　　　　　　if the statement does not agree with the writer；

NOT GIVEN　　if there is no information about this in the passage.

1. People with HIVwill eventually become AIDS patient.

2. Many people with HIV have no symptoms for several years.

3. If a person has an enlarged gland, he or she may be infected with HIV.

4. There are only three ways from which HIV can be transmitted.

5. Pregnant women who are infected with HIV risk passing the infection to the unborn fetus.

6. It is possible to be infected with HIV if people receive transplanted organ from infected people.

7. Doctors will not suggest people to take blood test if people have asmall chance of having been infected HIV.

8. People who are HIV positive need to have more blood tests every so often.

A2. The reading passage AIDS has six sections. Choose the most suitable heading for each section from the list of headings below. Write the appropriate letters（A-H）. Please note that there are more headings than you can use.

List of headings

A　What is the difference between HIV and AIDS?

B　The relationship between HIV and AIDS

C　Transmission of HIV

D　What is AIDS? What is HIV?

E　Blood test that measures HIV positive

F　Diagnosis of AIDS

G　Treatment for HIV/AIDS

H　Symptoms of early HIV infection

1. Section Ⅰ _____

2. Section Ⅱ _____

3. Section Ⅲ _____

4. Section Ⅳ _____

5. Section Ⅴ _____

6. Section Ⅵ _____

B1. Choose the appropriate words and fill in the blanks with their correct forms.

vulnerable	available	expose	symptom
pregnancy	transmit	infect	diagnose

1. Their cancers are not so clearly tied to radiation _____ .

2. The refugees, without a doubt, are the most _____ .

3. There is a risk of _____ of the virus between hypodermic users.

4. _____ diseases are spreading among many of the flood victims.

5. It would be wiser to cut out all alcohol during _____

6. Doctors examine their patients thoroughly in order to make a correct _____ .

7. Not enough data is _____ to scientists.

8. He has exhibited _____ of anxiety and overwhelming worry.

B2. Match the word with the meaning.

Word	Meaning
a. itchy	i. in the end; finally
b. symptom	ii. set of symptom which together indicate a particular disease
c. vulnerable	iii. having or producing irritation on the skin
d. ultimately	iv. gain by one's own ability, efforts, or behavior
e. syndrome	v. change in the body that indicates an illness
f. acquire	vi. be more likely to get a disease than other people, animals. or plants

B3. Study the following prefix and guess the meaning.

anti—against	antibody
ex—out	expose
sym—, syn—together, the same	syndrome

1. antipathy _____   2. antibacterial _____

3. antithesis _____   4. sympathy _____

5. synthesis _____   6. synonym _____

7. exclude _____   8. exhale _____

C1. Tick (√) the correct underlined verbs, and correct the verbs that are wrong.

I would like to be considered for your degree course in Dance, starting in September next year! I feel I am a good candidate for this course as I 1. have always been interested in dancing and even as a child I 2. have enjoyed dancing in my room. Your faculty has a good reputation and I would like to be part of it. As you 3. already saw in Section A of this application, I have a good academic record and I 4. just received the results of my recent exams, all of which 5. have been excellent.

   1. _____   2. _____   3. _____

4. _____ 5. _____

C2. Choose the best answer.

1. We _____ our new neighbours yet, so we don't know their names.

    A. don't meet   B. won't meet

    C. haven't met   D. hadn't met

2. The students _____ busily when Miss Brown went to get a book she _____ in her office.

    A. had written; left   B. were writing; has left

    C. had written; had left   D. were writing; had left

3. Mike _____ the bookshop. I have to wait for him.

    1. went to   B. was in

    C. has been to   D. has gone to

4. He kept look at her, wondering whether he _____ her somewhere else.

    A. saw   B. has seen

    C. sees   D. had seen

5. I _____ my aunt three times today, but her line was always busy.

    A. have phoned   B. phoned

    C. am phoning   D. will phone

C3. Translation

1. 这是我曾经看过的最好的一部电影。

2. 只是在我失明之后我才看透了他。

3. 约翰已经试过好多次了，因此他现在可以做得很好。

4. 自从 HIV 病毒被确认以来已经传遍了地球的每个角落。

5. HIV 检测有两个步骤，包括初筛试验和确认试验。

LISTENING

听力 A

Part A Listen to the first part of the report and choose the best answer to each of the following questions.

1. Who are not involved in preparing for the International AIDS Conference?

    A. Researchers   B. Activists

    C. The Obama Administration   D. Policy makers

2. Where will the next conference be held?

    A. Vietnam   B. Vienna

    C. Australia   D. America

3. What's the aim of America's National HIV/AIDS Strategy?

    A. To make sure infected patients get treatment within three months

B. To increase the treatment rate of the infected to 65 percent

C. To produce more effective medicines for the infected

D. To reduce new HIV infections by twenty-five percent within five years.

4. What's the percentage of Americans who discover they are infected and get treatment within three months?

　　A. 25 percent　　　　　　　　B. 50 percent

　　C. 65 percent　　　　　　　　D. 85 percent

5. How many people worldwide are living with the virus?

　　A. 33 million　　　　　　　　B. 30 million

　　C. Over 1 million　　　　　　D. None of the above

Part B　Listen to the second part of the report and fill in the blanks with what you have heard.

听力 B

1. Last week, government scientists in the United States ＿＿＿＿＿＿＿＿ of two antibodies that raise hopes for an AIDS vaccine. They say these antibodies can ＿＿＿＿＿＿＿＿ of all known strains of HIV. Antibodies are proteins that the body makes to help ＿＿＿＿＿＿＿＿ itself against infection.

2. Researchers made the discovery at the National Institute of Allergy and ＿＿＿＿＿＿＿＿ Diseases. The director of its Vaccine Research Center, Gary Nabel, says each antibody blocks the virus from ＿＿＿＿＿＿＿＿ white blood cells.

3. （GARY NABLE：）"It reacts with that region, it inactivates the virus and the virus never ＿＿＿＿＿＿＿＿ that it would otherwise infect."

4. The antibodies were discovered in a man, known as Donor 45, whose body produced them ＿＿＿＿＿＿＿＿. Patients with HIV must take medicine all their lives to prevent AIDS. ＿＿＿＿＿＿＿＿ are able to suppress the deadly virus in the body —— not a cure, but the next best thing.

5. In another development, the United Nations reported Tuesday that the number of young people ＿＿＿＿＿＿＿＿ in Africa is falling. The U. N. AIDS agency gives credit to better use of ＿＿＿＿＿＿＿＿ measures. It says young people in Africa are waiting longer to have sex. They are also having fewer sexual partners. And they are ＿＿＿＿＿＿＿＿ using condoms. As a result, the agency says HIV rates are falling in sixteen of the twenty-five ＿＿＿＿＿＿＿＿ countries in Africa.

书网融合······

微课 1　　　微课 2　　　微课 3　　　自测题

PPT

Unit 15 Arthritis

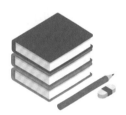

OBJECTIVES

When you have completed Unit 15, you will be able to

⊙ understand and identify professional terms related to arthritis.

⊙ communicate with the doctor about some typical symptoms properly.

⊙ skim the passage for main idea.

⊙ describe the symptoms, the causes and the control of arthritis.

⊙ obtain information about Arthritis by listening to the lecture.

⊙ master the structure "*as with*".

LEAD IN

Are you aware of the following symptoms in your joints? If you have more YES to the questions, you need to be careful! Arthritis is approaching you.

⊙ Joint pain

⊙ Joint swelling

⊙ Stiffness, especially in the morning

⊙ Warmth around a joint

⊙ Redness of the skin around a joint

⊙ Reduced ability to move the joint

会话

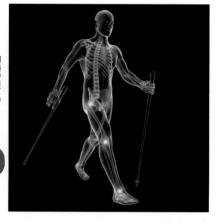

CONVERSATION

Sam and Jennifer are two American travelers in China. To have Chinese dishes, they need to learn how to use chopsticks. Here is a conversation between them. As a Chinese, do you believe in what they claimed?

Sam: It's a pain to learn how to use chopsticks. I just want to grab the food with my hands.

Jennifer: Oh I agree, it's not easy. By the way, have you ever heard of a study report on chopsticks and osteoarthritis?

Sam: No, I haven't. I cannot see the relationship between them.

Jennifer: You need to understand what osteoarthritis is to see the link.

Sam: I know what osteoarthritis is. Osteoarthritis is a disease of the joints caused by repeated use of particular joint. Normally the ends of bones are covered with a shock-absorber-like pad of springy cartilage. When cartilage wears down, bone end rubs against bone end on a joint, causing stiffness and often extreme pain.

Jennifer: Sam, you are almost an expert of osteoarthritis.

Sam: Don't flatter me. What does this have to do with chopsticks?

Jennifer: Now you are using chopsticks and in order to pinch two chopsticks together, do you have to put stress on the thumb and forefinger?

Sam: Oh, I am starting to see the relationship. Any repetitive motion involving the fingers can amplify the effects of naturally occurring cartilage decay.

Jennifer: Exactly. The thumb joint is the primary victim of chopstick use.

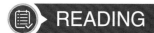

Sam: But we are just tourists who occasionally use chopsticks, we needn't worry about it.

Jennifer: Sure. Just imagine people in Asian countries make this motion every meal every day of their lives!

Sam: Oh, come on Jennifer. Let's stop worrying about the Asian people and their joint health. What we do should now is to finish our meal.

Jennifer: Ok, let's hurry up.

📖 READING

Arthritis

Pre – reading

Is it right to say arthritis occurs only in the elderly population?

Can you name some forms of arthritis?

For healthy joints, is exercise more important than rest?

While – reading

What Is Arthritis?

Arthritis is inflammation of one or more joints, which results in pain, swelling, stiffness, and limited movement. Arthritis comprises more than 100 different rheumatic disease and conditions, the most common of which is osteoarthritis.[1] Other frequently occurring forms of arthritis include rheumatoid arthritis, lupus, fibromyalgia, and gout.

Cause and Risk Factors

Arthritis involves the breakdown of cartilage. Cartilage normally protects the joint, allowing for smooth movement. Cartilage also absorbs shock when pressure is placed on the joint, like when you walk. Without the usual amount of cartilage, the bones rub together, causing pain, swelling, and stiffness.

You may have joint inflammation for a variety of reasons, including:

⊙ broken bone

⊙ infection (usually caused by bacteria or viruses)

⊙ an autoimmune disease (the body attacks itself because the immune system believes a body part is foreign)

⊙ general "wear and tear" on joints

Often, the inflammation goes away after the injury has healed, the disease is treated, or the infection has been cleared. With some injuries and diseases, the inflammation does not go away or destruction results in long-term pain and deformity. When this happens, you have chronic arthritis. Osteoarthritis is the most common type and is more likely to occur as you age. You may feel it in any of your joints, but most commonly in your hips, knees or fingers. Risk factors for osteoarthritis include:

⊙ being overweight

⊙ previously injuring the affected joint

⊙ using the affected joint in a repetitive action that puts stress on the joint (Baseball players, ballet dancers, and construction workers are all at risk).

Signs and Tests

First, your doctor will take a detailed medical history to see if arthritis or another musculoskeletal problem is the likely cause of your symptoms.

Next, a thorough physical examination may show that fluid is collecting around the joint. (This is called an "effusion".) The joint may be tender when it is gently pressed, and may be warm and red (especially in infectious arthritis and autoimmune arthritis). It may be painful or difficult to rotate the joints in some directions. This is known as "limited range of motion."

Tests vary depending on the suspected cause. They often include blood tests and joint X-rays. To check for infection and other causes of arthritis, joint fluid is removed from the joint with a needle and examined under a microscope.

Medication

Your doctor will choose from a variety of medications as needed. Generally, the first drugs to try are available without a prescription. These include: Acetaminophen (Tylenol)—recommended by the American College of Rheumatology and the American Geriatrics Society as first-line treatment for osteoarthritis. Aspirin, ibuprofen, or naproxen—these nonsteroidal anti-inflammatory (NSAID) drugs are often effective in combating arthritis pain. However, they have many potential risks, especially if used for a long time. They should not be taken in any amount without consulting your doctor.

Prescription medicines include:

Cyclooxygenase-2 (COX-2) inhititors; Corticosteroids ("steroids"); Disease-modifying anti-rheumatic drugs; Biologics; Immunosupressants.

It is very important to take your medications as directed by your doctor.

Treatment

Treatment of arthritis depends on the particular cause, which joints are affected, severity, and how the condition affects your daily activities.[2] Your age and occupation will also be taken into consideration when your doctor works with you to create a treatment plan.

If possible, treatment will focus on eliminating the underlying cause of the arthritis. However, the cause is NOT necessarily curable, as with osteoarthritis and rheumatoid arthritis.[3] Treatment, therefore, aims at reducing your pain and discomfort and preventing further disability.

It is possible to greatly improve your symptoms from osteoarthritis and other long-term types of arthritis without medications. In fact, making lifestyle changes without medications is preferable for osteoarthritis and other forms of joint inflammation. If needed, medications should be used in addition to lifestyle changes.

Exercise for arthritis is necessary to maintain healthy joints, relieve stiffness, reduce pain and fatigue, and improve muscle and bone strength. Your exercise program should be tailored to you as an individual.[4] Work with a physical therapist to design an individualized program, which should include: range of motion exercises for flexibility; strength training for muscle tone; and low-impact aerobic activity (also called endurance exercise).

Rest is just as important as exercise. Sleeping 8 to 10 hours per night and taking naps during the day can help you recover from a flare-up more quickly and may even help prevent exacerbations.

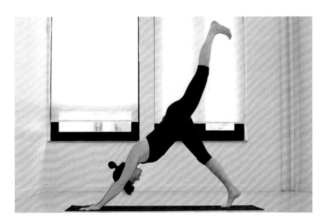

Notes

1. Arthritis comprises more than 100 different rheumatic disease and conditions, the most common of which is osteoarthritis.

"the most common of which" 中的 which 指代的是 "more than 100 different rheumatic disease and conditions", 当定语从句的主语是数词、形容词的最高级时, 一般只用 of whom 和 of which。这句话可译为: "关节炎包含有 100 多种各样的风湿性疾病和状况, 其中最普遍的就是骨关节炎。"

2. Treatment of arthritis depends on the particular cause, which joints are affected, severity, and how the condition affects your daily activities.

这句的谓语动词是 depend on, 意为 "取决于"。后面跟了语法结构各异的四个原因, 它们都是并列关系, 分别为: the particular cause; which joints are affected; severity; how the conditions affects your daily activities.

3. However, the cause is NOT necessarily curable, as with osteoarthritis and rheumatoid arthritis.

"as with" 表示 "正如, 和…一样", 这句话可译为: 然而, 正如骨关节炎和风湿性关节炎一样, 并不是所有的病因都是能治愈的。

4. Your exercise program should be tailored to you as an individual.

"be tailored to" 是表示 "量体裁衣, 个性制作"。此句意为 "你的训练计划也应该是针对你个体制定的。"

Glossary

Word	English definition	Example
absorb v.	suck or take up or in	Plants absorb carbon dioxide from the air and moisture from the soil
springy adj.	elastic; rebounds readily	Steam for about 12 minutes until the cake is springy to touch in the centre
flatter v.	praise somewhat dishonestly	I knew she was just flattering me
pinch v.	squeeze with the fingers	She pinched his arm as hard as she could
amplify v.	increase in size, volume or significance	The music was amplified with microphones
decay v.	undergo decay or decomposition	When not removed, plaque causes tooth decay and gum disease
comprise v.	include or contain; have as a component	The record is comprised of many old songs from the 1930's
result in	issue or terminate (in a specified way, state, etc.); end	This treatment could result in malformation of the arms
chronic adj.	being long-lasting and recurrent or characterized by long suffering	He has chronic bronchitis
tender adj.	sensitive and painful when it is touched	My tummy felt very tender
rotate v.	turn, as in a circle or cycle	Ballet dancers can rotate their legs by 90 degrees
suspect v.	imagine to be the case or true or probable	I suspect he is a fugitive
severity n.	used of the degree of something undesirable e. g. pain or weather	The criminal was punished with severity
occupation n.	the principal activity in your life that you do to earn money	He lost his occupation last month
Take…into consideration	give careful weighing of the reasons for or against something	When we plan an activity, we should take weather into consideration
eliminate v.	terminate, end, or take out	We must eliminate unnecessary steps and get directly to the point
underlying adj.	in the nature of something though not readily apparent	This word has its underlying meaning
relieve v.	provide physical relief, as from pain	Drugs can relieve much of the pain
fatigue n.	a feeling of extreme physical or mental tiredness	She continued to have severe stomach cramps, aches, fatigue, and depression
flexibility n.	the property of being flexible; easily bent or shaped	why do plant cells have this kind of flexibility
flare-up n.	a recurrence or an intensification	The flare-up of malaria killed many people
exacerbation n.	Increasing of the severity; aggravate	The exacerbation of the girl's disease worried her parents

Word	English definition	Chinese definition
joint *n.*	(anatomy) the point of connection between two bones or elements of a skeleton	关节
arthritis *n.*	inflammation of a joint or joints	关节炎
inflammation *n.*	a response of body tissues to injury or irritation; characterized by pain and swelling and redness and heat	炎症，发炎
swelling *n.*	an abnormal protuberance or localized enlargement	膨胀，肿胀
stiffness *n.*	the property of moving with pain or difficulty	僵硬
rheumatic *adj.*	of or pertaining to arthritis	风湿的
osteoarthritis *n.*	chronic breakdown of cartilage in the joints	骨关节炎
rheumatoid *adj.*	of or pertaining to arthritis	类风湿的
fibromyalgia *n.*	a rheumatoid disorder characterized by muscle pain and headaches	纤维性肌痛
deformity *n.*	an affliction in which some part of the body is misshapen or malformed	畸形
lupus *n.*	any of several forms of ulcerative skin disease	狼疮
gout *n.*	a painful inflammation of the big toe and foot caused by defects in uric acid metabolism resulting in deposits of the acid and its salts in the blood and joints	痛风
cartilage *n.*	tough elastic tissue; mostly converted to bone in adults	软骨
autoimmune *adj.*	of or relating to the immune response of the body against substance normally present in the body	自身免疫的
wear and tear	decrease in value of an asset due to obsolescence or use	磨损
musculoskeletal *adj.*	relating to muscles and skeleton	［解］肌（与）骨骼的
effusion *n.*	flow under pressure	流出；溢出
medication *n.*	something that treats or prevents or alleviates the symptoms of disease	药物
prescription *n.*	written instructions from a physician or dentist to a druggist concerning the form and dosage of a drug to be issued to a given patient	处方
acetaminophen *n.*	an analgesic for mild pain; also used as an antipyretic	对乙酰氨基酚

Word	English definition	Chinese definition
geriatrics *n.*	the branch of medical science that deals with diseases and problems specific to old people	老年病学
nonsteroidal *n. / adj.*	an organic compound that does no contain a steroid	非类固醇，非甾类化合物
cyclooxygenase *n.*	either of two related enzymes that control the production of prostaglandins and are blocked by aspirin	环氧酶
inhibitor *n.*	a substance that retards or stops an activity	抑制剂
corticosteroid *n.*	a steroid hormone produced by the adrenal cortex or synthesized; administered as drugs they reduce swelling and decrease the body's immune response	皮质类固醇；皮质甾
immunosuppressant *n.*	a substance that retards or stops an immuno activity	免疫抑制剂
aerobic *adj.*	depending on free oxygen or air	需氧的

Post – reading

A1. Complete the following " Arthritis At A Glance" with proper words：

Arthritis is 1 ＿＿＿＿＿＿ of one or more joints. It comprises more than 100 different rheumatic diseases and conditions, the most common of which is 2 ＿＿＿＿＿＿. Other frequently occurring forms of arthritis include rheumatoid arthritis, lupus, fibromyalgia, and gout. Common symptoms include pain, aching, 3 ＿＿＿＿＿＿, and swelling in or around the joints. Some forms of arthritis, such as rheumatoid arthritis and lupus, can affect multiple organs and cause widespread symptoms. A 4 ＿＿＿＿＿＿ is a medical arthritis expert. Although arthritis is more common among adults aged 65 years or older, people of all ages (including children) can be affected. Earlier and accurate diagnosis can help to prevent irreversible damage and 5 ＿＿＿＿＿＿. The treatment of arthritis is very 6 ＿＿＿＿＿＿ on the precise type of arthritis present. Treatments available include change of lifestyle, physical therapy, anti-inflammation medications, immune-altering medications, and surgical operations.

A2. Answer the following questions.

1. What is arthritis?

2. What are the reasons of joint inflammation?

3. What will happen to our bones if there is no usual amount of cartilage?

4. What is "limited range of motion"?

5. What are the factors influencing treatment of arthritis?

B1. Choose the appropriate words and fill in the blanks with their correct forms.

wear and tear	deform	preferable	exacerbate
pronounced	low-impact	individualize	tailor
prompt	alternative		

1. The ＿＿＿＿＿＿＿＿ design of this treadmill with cushioning can protect joints against injury.

2. Michael Horn says the laptops made it possible to truly ＿＿＿＿＿＿＿＿ the lessons.

3. Christine approaches him stealthily and snatches away his mask, revealing a hideously ＿＿＿＿＿＿＿＿ face.

4. She's so honey-lipped that she knows how to ＿＿＿＿＿＿＿＿ her words to please the ears of different people.

5. I couldn't afford the trip to Xinjiang, so I had no ＿＿＿＿＿＿＿＿ but to stay at home this vacation.

6. As I write this letter, I do not know that there is an opening at present, but here are my qualifications which ＿＿＿＿＿＿＿＿ me to make application now.

7. There was an even more ＿＿＿＿＿＿＿＿ link between regular dancing in three-inch heels and a reduced risk of knee problems.

8. But since it would be too much to discuss all seven plans at the same time, it is ＿＿＿＿＿＿＿＿ to stagger the airing of views and debates by the masses.

9. Because the grease was almost gone, the gears suffered form serious ＿＿＿＿＿＿＿＿ .

10. Some officials they are skeptical of a ban that would upset the powerful biotechnology industry and could ＿＿＿＿＿＿＿＿ tensions with important trading partners like the United States.

B2. Choose the best words for the following questions.

1. Fifty states ＿＿＿＿＿＿＿＿ the Unites States.

    A. include   B. comprise   C. comprise of   D. consist

2. The milk hug has been overturned, and I ＿＿＿＿＿＿＿＿ the cat.

    A. suspected   B doubted   C. think   D. confirmed

3. Stress and tiredness often ＿＿＿＿＿＿＿＿ a lack of concentration.

    A. result from   B. contribute   C. lead   D. result in

4. The dictator had ＿＿＿＿＿＿＿＿ all his political opponents.

    A. get rid of   B eliminated   C. destroyed   D. terminate

5. The ＿＿＿＿＿＿＿＿ assumption is that the amount of money available is limited.

    A. underlying   B. hidden   C. underground   D. fundamental

C1. **Complete each sentence using the best word（adjective or adverb form）from the box.**

usual（ly）	wonderful（ly）	heavy（ily）	strong（ly）
true（ly）	regular（ly）	common（ly）	genuine（ly）
bitter（ly）	high（ly）		

1. My maths teacher had a _____ influence on men when I was at school.

2. We used to do all the _____ things that children get up to!

3. My father and I see each other on a _____ basis.

4. When you live with someone you discover their _____ character.

5. When I didn't get into my preferred course, I was _____ disappointed.

6. It is a _____ mistake to think that you can study and work at the same time.

7. My trip to Macao was great fun and full of _____ surprises.

8. In Paris, we parked in a no-standing zone and got a _____ fine.

9. To be a vet, you'd need to have a _____ affection for animals.

C2. **Choose the best answer for the following questions.**

1. In actual fact he is ignorant on the subject. _____ he knows about it is out of date and inaccurate.

   A. What little　　　B. So much　　　C. How much　　　D. So little

2. Prof. Lee's book will show you _____ can be used in other contexts.

   A. that you have observed　　　　　B. that how you have onbserved

   C. how that you have observed　　　 D. how what you have observed

3. I will give this dictionary to _____ wants to have it.

   A. whoever　　　B. someone　　　C. whoever　　　D. anyone

4. They lost their way in the forest, and _____ made matters worse was that night began to fall.

   A. that　　　B. it　　　C. what　　　D. which

5. Although _____ happened in that developed country sounds like science fiction, it could occur elsewhere in the world.

   A. which　　　B. what　　　C. how　　　D. it

6. _____ is no reason for discharging her.

   A. Because she was a few minutes late

   B. Owing to a few minutes being late

   C. The fact that she was a few minutes late

   D. Being a few minutes late

7. Concerns were raised _____ witnesses might be encouraged to exaggerate their stories in court to ensure.

   A. what　　　B. when　　　C. which　　　D. that

8. _____ our team seems to lack at the moment is the determination _____ it will win.

    A. Whatever；that   B. What；that

    C. That；whether   D. Whether；that

C3. Translation

1. 关节炎会导致软骨的破坏。

2. 轻压关节时会感到疼痛。

3. 遵医嘱进行服药是非常重要的。

4. 泰诺是治疗骨关节炎的一线药物。

5. 休息和运动同等重要。

听力

LISTENING

You are going to hear a report on Finding New Ways to Treat Rheumatoid Arthritis. Refer to the listening and look at the statements below. Write

True   if the statement agrees with the listening material

False   if the statement does not agree with the listening material

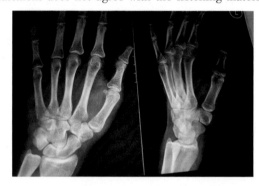

1. Women are four times more likely to get rheumatoid arthritis than men.

2. Rheumatoid arthritis is considered an autoimmune disease.

3. Professor Perlman believes the treatment could work in people.

4. Current treatments for rheumatoid arthritis do not have side effects.

5. According to Medline Plus Medical Encyclopedia，there are more than two hundred kinds of arthritis.

6. The most common form of arthritis is osteoarthritis.

书网融合……

微课1

微课2

微课3

自测题

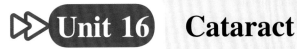 **Unit 16** **Cataract**

PPT

OBJECTIVES

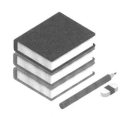

When you have completed Unit 16, you will be able to

⊙ understand and identify professional terms related to cataract.

⊙ communicate with the doctor about some typical symptoms properly.

⊙ skim the passage for main idea.

⊙ describe the symptoms, the causes and the control of cataract.

⊙ obtain information about cataract by listening to the lecture.

⊙ master the structure *"contrary to"*.

LEAD IN

Ben's father, Tom, always complains about his eyes.

"I do not see well enough to do my best at work."

"I need to drive, but there is too much glare from the sun or headlights."

"I do not see well enough to do the things I need to do at home."

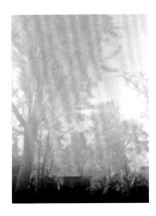 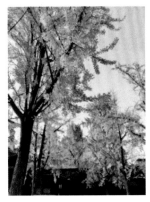 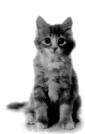 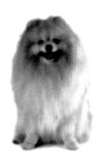

"I do not see well enough to do things I like to do (for example, read, watch TV, sew, take a walk, play cards or go out with friends.)"

"I am afraid I will bump into something or fall. "

"My glasses do not help me see well enough. "

"My glass number is changing very frequently. "

"My weak eyesight bothers me a lot. "

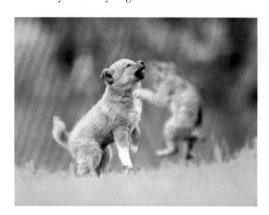
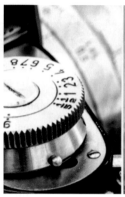
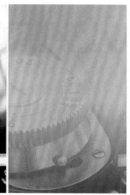

CONVERSATION

会话

Ben's father goes to a doctor about his eye sight.

Tom：Good morning, doctor.

Doctor：Good morning! What can I do for you?

Tom：I am having a problem with my eyes. My vision has been very poor lately. It's very blurred, and I've got to have a bright light to read anything these days.

Doctor：With the vision that you've got, are you able to do everything, or is it holding you back? Is your vision interfering with your lifestyle?

Tom：I'm not sure, Doctor.

Doctor：I see. Are you still having trouble with your diabetes?

Tom：Yes. But we are gradually getting it under control.

Doctor：I see. Then let's do an examination on your eyes.

(Fifteen minutes later)

Doctor：The problem is that you have a cataract. It's an opacity of the lens of the eye. It's often associated with diabetes or with getting older.

Tom：So doctor, how can we solve it?

Doctor：Surgery may be the best way to tackle it.

Tom：Surgery?

Doctor：Yep, and if I were you I wouldn't put off the decision because the sooner you have your surgery, the sooner you'll be able to get back your normal sight. You do have an early degree of cataract, but if it interferes with your ability to enjoy your life, we should consider operating.

Tom：Oh，then I'll make an appointment for the surgery.

Doctor：Ok.

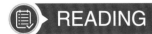 **READING**

Cataract

Pre – reading

What part of the body is affected if there is a cataract?

What are the symptoms?

How is it treated?

While – reading

What Is A Cataract?

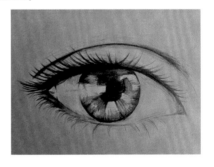

A cataract is a clouding of the lens in the eye that affects vision. Contrary to popular belief，cataract is not caused by eye strain or reading too much，but is a result of aging，injury，steroid use，exposure to UV light，smoking & diabetes. [1] Almost every person develops cataract changes as the eye ages. It is a natural process of eye aging. A cataract can occur in either or both eyes. It cannot spread from one eye to the other.

What Is a Lens?

The lens is a clear part of the eye that helps to focus light，or an image，on the retina. The retina is the light-sensitive tissue at the back of the eye. In a normal eye，light passes through the transparent lens to the retina. Once it reaches the retina，light is changed into nerve signals that are sent to the brain.

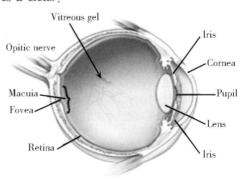

The lens must be clear for the retina to receive a sharp image. If the lens is cloudy from a cataract, the image you see will be blurred. When the blurring gets worse it is better to have the cloudy lensremoved by an operation and replaced by a clear artificial lens.[2]

Symptoms

The most common symptoms of a cataract are:

⊙ cloudy or blurry vision

⊙ colors seem faded

⊙ glare(Headlights, lamps, or sunlight may appear too bright. A halo may appear around lights).

⊙ poor night vision.

⊙ double vision or multiple images in one eye(This may clear as the cataract gets larger.)

⊙ frequent prescription changes in your eyeglasses or contact lens

These symptoms also can be a sign of other eye problems. If you have any of these symptoms, check with your eye care professional.

How Is It Detected?

Cataract is detected through a comprehensive eye exam that includes:

1. Visual acuity test. This eye chart test measures how well you see at various distances.

2. Dilated eye exam. Drops are placed in your eyes to widen, or dilate, the pupils. Your eye care professional uses a special magnifying lens to examine your retina and optic nerve for signs of damage and other eye problems. After the exam, your close-up vision may remain blurred for several hours.

3. Tonometry. An instrument measures the pressure inside the eye. Numbing drops may be applied to your eye for this test. Your eye care professional also may do other tests to learn more about the structure and health of your eye.

How Is a Cataract Detected?

The symptoms of an early cataract may be improved with new eyeglasses, brighter lighting, anti-glare sunglasses, or magnifying lenses. If these measures do not help, surgery is the only effective treatment. Surgery involves removing the cloudy lens and replacing it with an artificial lens.[3]

A cataract needs to be removed only when vision loss interferes with your everyday activities, such as driving, reading, or watching TV. You and your eye care professional can make this decision together. Once you understand the benefits and risks of surgery, you can make an informed decision about whether cataract surgery is right for you. In most cases, delaying cataract surgery will not cause long-term damage to your eye or make the surgery more difficult. You do not have to rush into surgery.

Sometimes a cataract should be removed even if it does not cause problems with your vision. For example, a cataract should be removed if it prevents examination or treatment of another eye problem, such as age-related macular degeneration or diabetic retinopathy. If your eye care professional finds a cataract, you may not need cataract surgery for several years. In fact, you might never need cataract surgery. By having your vision tested regularly, you and your eye care professional can discuss if and when you might need treatment.

If you choose surgery, your eye care professional may refer you to a specialist to remove the cataract.[4] If you have cataracts in both eyes that require surgery, the surgery will be performed on each eye at separate times, usually four to eight weeks apart.

Notes

1. Contrary to popular belief, a cataract is not caused by eye strain or reading too much, but is a result of aging, injury, steroid use, exposure to UV light, smoking and diabetes.

句中…not…but…连接两个并列谓语。短语"exposure to…"意为"暴露于……中"，如：Continuous exposure to sound above 80 decibels could be harmful. "contrary to"意为"与……相反"，例如：Contrary to what you might think, neither man was offended.

2. When the blurring gets worse it is better to have the cloudy lens removed by an operation and replaced by a clear artificial lens.

句型"it is better to do sth."意为"最好做……"此句型还可延展为"It is better to do …than to do…"表示"比起…来还是…"如：It is better to teach a man fish than to give him fish. （授之以鱼不如授之以渔）。短语"have the cloudy lens removed"为"have sth. done"结构，其主要意思有：

（1）（主语）请/派别人完成某事。

例：I had that door painted last week.

（2）（主语）完成某事（可能参与）。

例：They are going to have some trees planted.

（3）（主语）遭受某种不幸的情况。

例：I had my hat blown off.

3. Surgery involves removing the cloudy lens and replacing it with an artificial lens.

此句中"involve"一词为"包括,包含"之意。英文释义为"If a situation or activity involves something, that thing is a necessary part or consequence of it."例如：A retrofit may involve putting in new door jambs.（房子翻新可能需要安装新的门框。）

4. If you choose surgery, your eye care professional may refer you to a specialist to remove the cataract.

"refer …to…"此句中的意思为"把…推荐给…"如：I referred her to Tom for further information.

Glossary

Word	English definition	Example
exposure *n.*	vulnerability to the elements; to the action of heat or cold or wind or rain	Exposure to lead is known to damage the brains of young children
transparent *adj.*	able to be seen through with clarity	The insect's wings are almost transparent
blur *v.*	become glassy; lose clear vision	Her eyes, behind her glasses, began to blur
opacity *n.*	the quality of being difficult to see through	Opacity of the eye lens can be induced by deficiency of certain vitamins
tackle *v.*	deal with a difficult problem or task in a very determined or efficient way	The first reason to tackle these problems is to save children's lives
artificial *adj.*	not arising from natural growth or characterized by vital processes	Our range of herbal teas contain no preservatives, colourings or artificial flavourings
fade *v.*	become less clearly visible or distinguishable; disappear gradually or seemingly	All color fades-especially under the impact of direct sunlight
glare *n.*	great brightness	Special-purpose glasses reduce glare
detect *v.*	discover or determine the existence, presence, or fact of	We are trying to detect and understand how the climates change
comprehensive *adj.*	including all or everything	There are much brighter prospects for a comprehensive settlement than before
acuity *v.*	sharpness of vision; the visual ability to resolve fine detail (usually measured by a Snellen chart)	We work on improving visual acuity
measure *v.*	have certain dimensions	The cushions, shown left, measure 20×12 inches and cost $39. 95
numbing *adj.*	causing numbness or insensitivity	Watching television had a numbing effect on his mind
dilate *v.*	become wider	At night, the pupils dilate to allow in more light
magnify *v.*	increase in size, volume or significance	He tried to magnify the part he played in the battle
optic *adj.*	relating to or using sight	The reason for this is that the optic nerve is a part of the brain
interfere *v.*	come between so as to be hindrance or obstacle	Smoking and drinking interfere with your body's ability to process oxygen

Word	English definition	Example
informed *adj.*	having much knowledge or education	According to informed sources, those taken into custody include at least one major-general

Word	English definition	Chinese definition
cataract *n.*	clouding of the natural lens of the eye	白内障
diabetes *n.*	a medical condition in which someone has too much sugar in their blood	糖尿病
lens *n.*	the part behind the pupil that focuses light and helps you to see clearly	晶状体
eye strain	If you suffer from eye strain, you feel pain around your eyes or at the back of your eyes, because you are very tired or should be wearing glasses.	眼疲劳
steroid *n.*	any of several fat-soluble organic compounds having as a basis 17 carbon atoms in four rings	甾类化合物，类固醇
retina *n.*	the light-sensitive membrane covering the back wall of the eyeball; it is continuous with the optic nerve	视网膜
tissue *n.*	a part of an organism consisting of an aggregate of cells having a similar structure and function	组织
halo *n.*	an indication of radiant light drawn around the head of a saint	光晕
tonometry *n.*	a method for measuring intraocular pressure (IOP) and detecting glaucoma	眼压测量法
macular degeneration	a common, painless eye condition in which the central portion of the retina deteriorates and does not function adequately	黄斑部退化
retinopathy *n.*	a pathological disorder of the retina	视网膜病

Post – reading

A1. True/False/Not Given

Refer to the passage and look at the statements below. Write

True　　　　if the statement agrees with the writer;

False　　　　if the statement does not agree with the writer;

NOT GIVEN if there is no information about this in the passage.

1. A cataract is caused by reading too much.

2. A cataract only occurs in one eye.

3. The retina is light-sensitive and locates behind the eye.

4. In the dilated eye exam, a special magnifying lens is used to exam the retina and optic nerve.

5. The early cataract cannot be improved.

A2. Scan and complete the sentences.

1. A cataract is a result of aging, injury, _____ use, _____ to UV light, smoking and _____.

2. When the _____ gets worse it is better to have _____ removed by an operation and _____ by a clear _____ lens.

3. A _____ may appear around lights.

4. Drops are placed in your eyes to _____, or _____, the _____.

5. A cataract should be removed if it prevents _____ or _____ of another eye problem, such as age-related _____ or _____.

B1. Choose the appropriate words and fill in the blanks with their correct forms.

transparent	blur	artificial	fade
glare	comprehensive	dilate	interfere

1. The Rough Guide to Nepal is a _____ guide to the region.

2. Alexander wasn't going to let a lack of space _____ with his plans.

3. The adhesive tape Monica chose was _____ so that when she repaired her torn notebook, the teacher could still read the homework exercises beneath it.

4. Organic food is unadulterated food produced without _____ ingredients, chemicals or pesticides.

5. This creates a spectrum of colours at the edges of objects which _____ the image.

6. Exercise _____ blood vessels on the surface of the brain.

7. The colours gently _____ each time you wash the shirt.

8. His glasses magnified his irritable _____ eyes.

B2. Match according to the explanations.

Word	Explanation
a. cataract	i.
b. steroid	ii. a light-sensitive layer of tissue, lining the inner surface of the eye

续表

Word	Explanation
c. retina	iii.
d. macular	iv. the substance along with phospholipids functions as components of cell membranes. Cholesterol ones decrease membrane fluidity
e. tonometry	v.

B3. Guess meaning from prefix and suffix.

retino-视网膜　retinodialysis 视网膜分离

－pathy：Latin suffix＝abnormality or disease　psychopathy 心理病变　electropathy 电疗法

pathology ＿＿＿＿＿＿　　　　zoopathology ＿＿＿＿＿＿

neuropathy ＿＿＿＿＿＿　　　　hydropathy ＿＿＿＿＿＿

C1. Fill in the blanks with the proper forms, including the "to" stem for infinitives if necessary.

1. A computer does only what people have it ＿＿＿＿＿＿（do）.

2. Who did you have ＿＿＿＿＿＿（paint）the wall yesterday?

3. I'm sorry I can't help you because I have a lot of letters ＿＿＿＿＿＿（answer）.

4. The villagers are going to have a new bridge ＿＿＿＿＿＿（build）over the river.

5. Who allowed the candle ＿＿＿＿＿＿（burn）throughout the whole night?

6. What have they needed ＿＿＿＿＿＿（do）to stop the pollution from the chemical works?

7. Who had the teacher assigned ＿＿＿＿＿＿（clean）the blackboard?

C2. Multiple choice

1. —Some of the plastic bags can't ＿＿＿＿＿＿ after June 1.

—Yes，people will use environmental bags instead.

A. use   B. be use   C. be used   D. are used

2. —There is a lot of wind in North China.

—Well，more trees ＿＿＿＿＿＿ every year to stop the wind.

A. must be planted   B. can planted   C. should planted

C3. Complete the sentences according to the requirements.

1. Teenagers should be allowed to play with friends at night.（改为否定句）

Teenagers ＿＿＿＿＿＿ to play with friends at night.

2. The flowers must be watered once a day.（改为一般疑问句）

＿＿＿＿＿＿ the flowers ＿＿＿＿＿＿ once a day?

3. Should the classroom be cleaned on time?（作肯定回答）

＿＿＿＿＿＿，＿＿＿＿＿＿.

4. Parents should allow children to choose their clothes.（改为被动语态）

Children ＿＿＿＿＿＿ to choose their clothes.

5. The young tree can be planted now.（改为主动语态）

We ＿＿＿＿＿＿ the young tree now.

C4. Translation

1. 有可靠证据表明日光曝晒与皮肤癌之间有联系。

2. 与通常的看法相反，适度的运动事实上会降低食欲。

3. 料理好厨房需要把一切都安排得规规矩矩，且要讲求速度。

4. 老师叫我去查第三章。

5. 白内障通常和糖尿病以及衰老有关。

LISTENING

听力

Part A   You are going to hear a brief introduction to cataract. Refer to the listening and look at the statements below. Write

True   if the statement agrees with the listening material

False   if the statement does not agree with the listening material

1. The lens cannot change its shape.

2. The earliest cataract surgery was done by Indians.

3. The second discovery is that the lens includes four layers.

4. In modern surgery we pull out the cloudy things and inject a plastic lens.

5. The lens in the fish eye moves back and forth.

Part B   Complete the sentences.

1. Well，let's take an eye model and some more videos. Take the model，open it up and look inside，we have a little _____ inside there，which are called the lens. The lens is _____ . It can change shape and help do a lot of things，like focusing. A cataract is that the lens becomes cloudy and that cloudy lens causes _____ .

2. In modern cataract surgery，they will take _____ ，stick to that cataract lens，break this lens and pull the entire cataract out.

3. Modern surgery has two discoveries，one is _____ and the second one is the discovery that the lens，that cloudy cataract，is not a single piece. It is more like peanut M&m in the sense that it has three layers. And this three layers help us change our surgery. The three layers are _____ （outside），_____ （between）and _____ （in the middle）.

4. Here is what we have done in modern surgery. We make a very small _____ ，and we take a little bit circle off，and then we break _____ and break up the peanut，we got all the peanut out，then move out the cortex. At last，we inject a new plastic lens.

5. There are some new technologies now. The first one is _____ . The surface is supposed to be round，like a basketball，however in the _____ ；the surface of the eye is more like a football. There is another way called _____ . One of the things we can do is go to the sea because there is a wide variety of eyes in the animal kingdom. In fact，we look at the fish. The four-eye fish is unique that the lens in their eyes look like _____ ，which is called _____ ，allowing them to see on top and things under water.

书网融合……

▶▶ Appendix 1　Glossary

A

abdominal［æbˈdɔminl］　adj. 腹部的

absenteeism［æbsənˈtiːizəm］　n. 旷工；旷课

absorb［əbˈzɔːb］　vt. 吸收；吸引

accumulate［əˈkjuːmjəleɪt］　v. 积累；增加；聚集

acetaminophen［ə,siːtəˈmɪnəfen］　n. 对乙酰氨基酚

acidic［əˈsidik］　adj. 酸的；酸性的

acuity［əˈkjuːɪtɪ］　n. 敏锐；尖锐；剧烈

acute［əˈkjuːt］　adj. 急性的

address［əˈdres］　vt. 把注意力集中于（某问题）；写地址；演说；称呼 n. 地址

aerobic［eəˈrəubɪk］　adj. 需氧的

aggregate［ˈægrigət］　vt. 使聚集，使积聚

allergen［ˈælədʒən］　n. 过敏原

alter［ˈɔːltə］　vt. 改变

alternate［ˈɔːltəːnət］　v. 交替；轮流

amplify［ˈæmplɪfaɪ］　vt. 放大

amputation［ˌæmpjʊˈteɪʃn］　n. 切断；＜医＞截肢（术）；切除；删除

androgen［ˈændrədʒ(ə)n］　n. 雄性激素；男性荷尔蒙

anemia［əˈniːmiːə］　n. 贫血症；无活力；无生气

angina［ænˈdZainə］　n. 心绞痛

angioplasty［ˈændZiəuplæsti］　n. 血管成形术

antacids［æntˈæsidz］　n. 解酸剂

antibiotics［æntɪbaɪˈɒtɪks］　n. 抗生素；抗生学

antibody［ˈæntɪbɒdɪ］　n. 抗体

anticoagulants［ænti:kəˈʊægjʊlənts］　n. ［医］抗凝［血］剂，抗凝［血］的

antihistamine［æntiˈhistəmiːn］　n. 抗组胺药

antioxidant［ˌæntiˈɒksɪdənt］　n. 抗氧化剂；硬化防止剂

approximately［əˈprɒksɪmətli］　adv. 近似地，大约

argumentative［ˌaːgjuˈmentətiv］　adj. 好辩的，争论的

arthritis［aːˈθraɪtɪs］　n. 关节炎

artificial［aːtɪˈfiʃ(ə)l］　adj. 人工的

assignment ［ə'saɪnm(ə)nt］　　n. 分配；任务；作业；功课

asthma ［'æsmə］　　n. 哮喘

atherosclerosis ［ˌæθərəʊskliˈrəʊsis］　　n. 动脉粥样硬化

autoimmune ［ˌɔːtəʊɪˈmjuːn］　　adj. 自身免疫的

B

bacteria ［bæk'tɪərɪə］　　n. 细菌（bacterium 的复数）

barium enema ［'beərɪəm 'enəmə］　　n. 钡灌肠

biopsies ［'baɪɒpsi］　　n. 活组织检查

bladder ［'blædə］　　n. 膀胱；囊状物

blocked ［blɒkt］　　adj. 堵塞的；被封锁的 v. 阻塞（block 的过去分词）

blur ［blɜː］　　vi. 沾上污迹；变模糊

blurred ［bləːd］　　adj. 模糊的；难辨的

blurry ［'blɜːri］　　adj. 模糊的；污脏的；污斑的

bowel ［'baʊəl］　　n. 肠

broccoli ［'brɒkəli］　　n. 西兰花；花椰菜

bronchial ［'brɒŋkɪəl］　　adj. 支气管的

bruising ［'bruːzɪŋ］　　adj. 殊死的；十分激烈的 v. 擦伤（bruise 现在分词形式）

bulge ［bʌldʒ］　　n. 膨胀；凸出部分；暴涨；突增 v. 凸出；膨胀；急增

bypass ［baipaːs］　　n. 旁道，支路［医］导管

C

calories ［'kælərɪz］　　n. 卡路里

cantaloupe ［'kæntəluːp］　　n. 罗马甜瓜；香瓜；哈密瓜

carbohydrate ［ˌkɑːbəʊ'haɪdreɪt］　　n. 碳水化合物；糖类；淀粉质或糖类食物

cardiovascular ［ˌkɑːdiəʊ'væskjələ(r)］　　adj. 心血管的

cartilage ［'kɑːt(ɪ)lɪdʒ］　　n. 软骨

cataract ［'kætərækt］　　n. 白内障

categorized ［'kætəgəraɪz］　　v. 把…归类；把…列作（categorize 过去式和过去分词）

causal ［'kɔːz(ə)l］　　adj. 因果关系的；有原因的

characterized ［'kærəktəraɪz］　　adj. ［医］具有特征的 v. 是…的特征（characterize 过去式和过去分词）

chill ［tʃɪl］　　n. 寒冷；寒意

chlordiazepoxide ［klɔːdaieizi'pɒksaid］　　n. 甲氨二氮䓬，利眠宁

cholesterol ［kə'lestərɔl］　　n. 胆固醇

chronic ［'krɒnɪk］　　adj. 慢性的；长期的

chug ［tʃʌg］　　v. 一口气喝完；发出轧轧声

cirrhosis［sə'rəusis］　n. <医 >肝硬化；硬化

citrus［'sɪtrəs］　n.［植］柑橘属果树；柠檬；柑橘

clonazepam［kləu'nəzpæm］　n.［化］氯硝西泮

clot［klɔt］　n. 凝块，血块

colon［'kəulən］　n. 结肠

comedo［'kɒmɪdəu］　n. 粉刺；面疱

comedogenic［kɔmi'dəudʒenik］　adj. 易生黑头粉刺的

complication［kɔmpli'keiʃn］　n. 并发症

comprehensive［ˌkɑːmprɪ'hensɪv］　adj. 综合的；广泛的

comprise［kəm'praɪz］　vt. 包含；由…组成

compromise［'kɔmprəmaiz］　vi. 妥协，退让

condiment［'kɔndimənt］　n. 调味品，佐料

consume［kən'sjuːm］　vt. 消耗；耗尽；吃光

consumption［kən'sʌmpʃn］　n. 消耗；肺病

coricidin［'kɔrisidin］　n. 柯利西锭（抗感冒药）

coronary［'kɔrənri］　adj. 冠状的；冠状动脉或静脉的 n. 冠状动脉

correlate［'kɔrəleit］　v. 使相互关联

corrode［kə'rəud］　v. 腐蚀；损害

corticosteroid［kɔtikəu'stiərɔid］　n. & adj. 皮质甾类（的），皮质类固醇（的）

cramp［kræmp］　n. 痛性痉挛，抽筋

cranberry［'krænb(ə)rɪ］　n. 蔓越橘

critical［'krɪtɪk(ə)l］　adj. 决定性的；评论的

cuff［kʌf］　n. 护腕；袖口

cyclooxygenase［ˌsaikləu'ɔksidʒineis］　n. 环氧酶

cystitis［sɪ'staɪtɪs］　n. 膀胱炎

D

dander［'dændə］　n. 头皮屑

decay［dɪ'kei］　vi. 衰退，腐烂

deficiency［dɪ'fɪʃnsi］　n. 缺乏；不足；缺点；缺陷；不足额

deformity［dɪ'fɔːmɪtɪ］　n. 畸形；畸形的人或物

density［'densɪtɪ］　n. 密度

destabilize［ˌdiː'steɪbəlaɪz］　v. 使打破平衡；使不稳定；使动摇

detect［dɪ'tekt］　vt. 察觉；发现；探测

deterioration［diˌtiəriə'reiʃn］　n. 恶化；退化

detoxification［diːˌtɔksifi'keiʃn］　n. 解毒，去毒作用

detrimental［ˌdetri'mentl］　adj. 有害的；不利的

dextromethorphan［dekstrəumi；ˈθɔːfn］　　n. 右美沙芬（镇咳药）

diabetes［ˌdaɪəˈbiːtiːz］　　n. 糖尿病

diabetic［ˌdaɪəˈbetɪk］　　adj. 糖尿病的 n. 糖尿病患者

diagnosis［ˌdaɪəgˈnəusɪs］　　n. 诊断

diarrhea［daɪəˈrɪə］　　n. 腹泻 adj. 腹泻的

diastolic［ˈdaɪəˈstɔlik］　　adj. 心脏舒张的

dilate［daɪˈleɪt］　　vt. &vi. 扩大；膨胀

discomfort［disˈkʌmfət］　　n. 不安；不舒适；不方便

disfigure［dɪsˈfɪgə］　　v. 使变丑；损毁…的外形；使大为减色

disorder［dɪsˈɔːdə］　　n. 混乱；骚乱 v. 使失调；扰乱

dissolve［dɪˈzɒlv］　　v. 溶解；融化；分裂；分解

distinguish［diˈstiŋgwiʃ］　　v. 区别；辨认

duodenum［djuːəˈdiːnəm］　　n. 十二指肠

duration［djuˈreiʃn］　　n. 持续，持续的时间

dysthymia［disˈθaimiə］　　n. 精神抑郁（症）

E

effusion［ɪˈfjuːʒ(ə)n］　　n. 渗出；泻出；渗漏物

elevated［ˈeliveitid］　　adj. 升高的；高层的；高尚的

eliminate［ɪˈlɪmɪneɪt］　　vt. 消除；排除

employ［imˈplɔi］　　vt. 利用，雇用

enamel［ɪˈnæml］　　n. 搪瓷；珐琅；指甲油 v. 给…上珐琅；在…涂瓷漆

encompass［inˈkʌmpəs］　　vt. 围绕；包含或包括某事物

end-stage renal disease［医］终末期肾脏疾病；晚期肾病

endoscopy［enˈdɔskəpi］　　n. ［医］内诊镜检查

engage in 参加，经营，忙于做某事

episode［ˈepisəud］　　n. 插曲；片段；一段经历

erosion［iˈrəuʒn］　　n. 腐蚀；减少，流失

esophagus［iˈsɔfəgəs］　　n. 食管

essential［iˈsenʃl］　　adj. 必要的；本质的；基本的 n. 必需品；基本要素

exacerbate［igˈzæsəbeit］　　vt. 使恶化；使加重

exacerbation［ek,sæsəˈbeiʃən］　　n. 恶化；激怒；增剧

exceed［ikˈsiːd］　　vt. 超过；超越；胜过 vi. 突出，领先

excessive［ɪkˈsesɪv］　　adj. 过多的；过分的；过度的；极度的；过逾

excrete［ikˈskriːt］　　vt. 排泄；分泌

expose［ɪkˈspəuz；ek－］　　vt. 揭露，揭发；使曝光；显示

exposure［ɪkˈspəuʒə；ek－］　　n. 暴露；曝光；揭露；陈列

extract ['ekstrækt]　vt. &n. 提取；提取物

F

fade [feɪd]　vi. 褪色；凋谢；逐渐消失

fast [fɑ:st]　v. 禁食；（尤指）斋戒 adj. 快的

fatigue [fə'ti:g]　n. &adj. 疲劳；疲乏 v. 使疲劳；使疲乏

fatty ['fæti]　adj. 油腻的；配胖的；多脂肪的 n. 胖子

fecal impaction ['fi:kl im'pækʃən]　n. 粪便嵌塞

feverish ['fi:v(ə)rɪʃ]　adj. 发热的；极度兴奋的

fibromyalgia [,faibrəumai'ældʒi:ə]　n. 纤维肌痛；纤维组织肌痛

flatter ['flætə]　v. 奉承；谄媚；使高兴

flexibility [,fleksɪ'bɪlɪtɪ]　n. 灵活性；弹性；适应性

folate ['fəuleit]　n. 叶酸

fortified ['fɔ:tɪfaɪd]　adj. 加强的 v. 筑防御工事于（fortify 过去式和过去分词）；增强

G

gangrene ['gæŋgri:n]　n. 坏疽 vi. 生坏疽；腐败

gastric ['gæstrik]　adj. 胃的

gastrointestinal [gæstrəuin'testinl]　adj. 胃肠的

geriatrics [dʒerɪ'ætrɪks]　n. 老年病学；老年病人

gestation [dʒe'steɪʃn]　n. 怀孕；怀孕期；构思；酝酿；孕育（过程）

gland [glænd]　n. 腺

glare [gleə]　n. 刺眼；耀眼的光

glaze [gleiz]　vi. （目光）变得呆滞无神

glucose ['glu:kəus]　n. [化] 葡萄糖；右旋糖

glycemic [glɪ'semɪk]　adj. 血糖的

gout [gaut]　n. 痛风

graft [grɑ:ft]　vi. & vt. 移植，嫁接

guarantee [,gærən'ti:]　n. 保证，保证书；抵押品 vt. 保证，担保

guava ['gwɑ:və]　n. 番石榴

guzzle ['gʌzl]　v. 狂饮；大量消耗

H

hair follicles ['fɒlɪk(ə)l]　n. 毛囊

hallucination [hə,lu:si'neiʃn]　n. 错觉；幻觉

halo ['heɪləu]　n. 光环；荣光

handle〔'hændl〕 vi. & vt. 操作，处理，管理

heredity〔hɪ'redɪtɪ〕 n. 遗传；遗传性

hormone〔'hɔːməʊn〕 n. 激素；荷尔蒙

hygiene〔'haidʒiːn〕 n. 卫生，卫生学；保健法

hyperglycemia〔ˌhaɪpəglaɪ'siːmɪə〕 n. 多糖症；高血糖症

hypertension〔ˌhaipə'tenʃn〕 n. 高血压

hyperthyroidism〔ˌhaɪpə'θaɪrɔɪdɪzəm〕 n. 甲状腺功能亢进

hypoglycemia〔ˌhaɪpəʊglaɪ'siːmɪə〕 n. 血糖过低；低血糖症

I

identify〔ai'dentifai〕 vi. & vt. 确定；识别

immune〔ɪ'mjuːn〕 adj. 免疫的；有免疫力的

immunosuppressant〔ˌɪmjʊnəʊsə'presənt〕 n. 免疫抑制剂

immunosuppressive〔i'mjuːnəʊsə'presiv〕 adj. 抑制免疫反应的

impaired〔im'peəd〕 adj. 受损的；不匹配的，不适合的

impede〔ɪm'piːd〕 v. 阻碍；妨碍；阻止

in a row –连；接连

indigestion〔indi'dʒestʃən〕 n. 消化不良

infect〔ɪn'fekt〕 vt. 感染，传染

infection〔ɪn'fekʃ(ə)n〕 n. 感染；传染；影响；传染病

inflamed〔ɪn'fleɪmd〕 adj. 发炎的；红肿的 v. 使发炎（inflame 过去分词）；激起

inflammation〔ɪnflə'meɪʃ(ə)n〕 n. 炎症；发炎

inflammatory〔in'flæmətri〕 adj. 发炎的；炎症的

informed〔ɪn'fɔːmd〕 adj. 消息灵通的；见多识广的

infrequent〔in'friːkwənt〕 adj. 不频发的；不常见的

inhale〔in'heil〕 v. 吸入

inheritance〔in'heritəns〕 n. 继承；遗传

inhibitor〔ɪn'hɪbɪtə〕 n. 抑制剂

initiate〔i'niʃieit〕 v. 开始；启蒙

inordinate〔in'ɔdinət〕 adj. 无节制的；过度的

insomnia〔ɪn'sɒmnɪə〕 n. ［医］失眠；失眠症

insulin〔'ɪnsjəlɪn〕 n. 胰岛素

intake〔'inteik〕 n. 吸入；摄入

intentionally〔in'tenʃənəli〕 adv. 有意地；故意地

interfere〔ɪntə'fɪə〕 vi&vt. . 干涉；妨碍；打扰

interfere with 干预；阻挠

intestine〔ɪn'testɪn〕 n. 肠

intoxicate［inˈtɔksikeit］ vt. 使喝醉；使陶醉；使激动不已

iodine［ˈaɪədiːn］ n. ＜化＞碘

irritability［ˌɪrɪtəˈbɪlɪtɪ］ n. 易怒；过敏性；兴奋性；感应性

irritable［ˈiritəbl］ adj. 易怒的；急躁的

irritation［ɪrɪˈteɪʃn］ n. 刺激；激怒，恼怒，生气

isotretinoin［aɪsəʊtrəˈtɪnəʊɪn］ n.（用来治疗严重痤疮的）异维 A 酸

itchy［ˈɪtʃɪ］ adj. 发痒的；渴望的

J

joint［dʒɔɪnt］ n. 关节；接缝；接合处

juvenile［ˈdʒuːvənaɪl］ adj. 少年的；幼稚的；年少无知的 n. 青少年，雏鸟

K

kidney［ˈkidni］ n. 肾，肾脏

kiwi［ˈkiːwiː］ n. ［植］猕猴桃；奇异果

L

laxative［ˈlæksətiv］ n. 泻药

lean［liːn］ adj. 瘦的；贫瘠的

lens［lenz］ n. 透镜，镜头，晶状体

libido［liˈbiːdəʊ］ n. 本能冲动，性欲

ligament［ˈlɪɡəmənt］ n. 纽带；［解］韧带

lump［lʌmp］ n. 肿块 v. 结成块；成团 adj. 成团的；成块的

lupus［ˈluːpəs］ n. 狼疮

M

magnify［ˈmæɡnɪfaɪ］ v. 放大

maintain［meɪnˈteɪn］ v. 保持；保养；坚持；固执己见

manic［ˈmænik］ adj. 躁狂的，患躁狂病的；

manifest［ˈmænifest］ vt. 显示，表明，使显现

measure［ˈmeʒə］ vt. ＆n. 测量；措施

medication［mediˈkeɪʃ(ə)n］ n. 药物；药物治疗；药物处理

menstrual［ˈmenstruəl］ adj. 月经的；每月的

metabolic［ˌmetəˈbɒlɪk］ adj. 新陈代谢的；变化的

metabolism［məˈtæbəlɪzəm］ n. 新陈代谢；代谢作用

minimize［ˈminimaiz］ vt. 变到最小，降到最低

misconception［mɪskənˈsepʃ(ə)n］ n. 误解；错觉；错误想法

mite ［maɪt］ n. 小虫

moderation ［ˌmɔdə'reiʃn］ n. 适度；自我节制；稳定

moisture ［'mɔɪstʃə］ n. 水分；湿度；潮湿

mould ［məʊld］ n. 霉菌

musculoskeletal ［ˌmʌskjʊləʊ'skelɪt(ə)l］ adj. 肌（与）骨骼的

N

narcotic ［nɑː'kɔtik］ adj. 麻醉的；有麻醉作用的

negative ［'negətiv］ adj. 消极的，否认的

neuropathy ［ˌnjʊə'rɒpəθɪ］ n. 神经病

neutralize ［'njuːtrəlaiz］ v. 使中立；中和

nicotinamide ［nɪkə'tɪnəmaɪd］ n. 烟酰胺；烟碱；尼克酰胺

nicotine ［'nikətiːn］ n. 尼古丁；

nitrate ［'naitreit］ n. 硝酸盐；硝酸酯

nodule ［'nɒdjuːl］ n. （尤指植物上的）节结；小瘤

nonsteroidal ［ˌnɔnstə'rɔidəl］ n. /adj. 非类固醇，非甾类化合物

numbing ［'nʌmɪŋ］ adj. 麻木的；失去知觉的

nutrition ［nju'trɪʃn］ n. 营养学；营养品；营养；滋养；食物

O

occupation ［ɒkjʊ'peɪʃ(ə)n］ n. 职业；占有

onset ［'ɒnset］ n. 攻击；袭击；开始；动手；［医］发病

opacity ［ə(ʊ)'pæsɪtɪ］ n. 不透明；不传导；暧昧

ophthalmopathy ［ɒf'θælməʊpəθɪ］ n. ［医］眼病

opportunistic ［ɒpətjuː'nɪstɪk］ adj. 机会主义的；投机取巧的

optic ［'ɒptɪk］ adj. 光学的；视觉的

organic ［ɔː'gænɪk］ adj. 有机（体）的；有组织的；系统的；器官的；根本的

osteoarthritis ［ˌɒstɪəʊɑː'θraɪtɪs］ n. 骨关节炎

P

pacnes n. 痤疮丙酸杆菌 propionibacterium acnes 缩写

palpitations ［ˌpælpɪ'teɪʃnz］ n. 心悸（palpitation 的名词复数）

pancreas ［'pæŋkriəs］ n. <解剖>胰；胰腺

papaya ［pə'paɪə］ n. 番木瓜树；番木瓜果

pee ［piː］ n. /v. 尿；撒尿

peptic ulcer ［'peptik 'ʌlsə］ n. 消化性溃疡

perforation ［pəːfə'reiʃn］ n. 孔；穿孔

periodic [ˌpiəri'ɔdik]　　adj. 定期的；　间歇的

persistent [pə'sistənt]　　adj. 坚持的；连续的

perspiration [ˌpɜːspə'reiʃn]　　n. 汗；汗水；出汗；流汗

pickle ['pikl]　　vt. 腌渍（泡菜等）n. 泡菜；腌制食品

pimple [pim'pəl]　　n. 丘疹，面疱

pinch [pin(t)ʃ]　　v. 捏，夹

plaque [plæk]　　n. [医] 血小板

pollen ['pɔlən]　　n. [植] 花粉

polydipsia [ˌpɒli'dipsiə]　　n. 烦渴

polyphagia [pɒli'feidʒiə]　　n. 多食症；杂食性

polyuria ['pɒli'jəriə]　　n. 多尿（症）

poop [puːp]　　n. / vi. 排便

positive ['pɒzitiv]　　adj. 阳性的

postpone [pə'spəʊn]　　vi. & vt. 延缓；延缓发作

pound [paʊnd]　　n. 磅；英镑；重击声 v. 连续重击；（心脏）狂跳

predict [pri'dikt]　　v. 预言；预测；预示；预告

pregnancy ['pregnənsi]　　n. 怀孕

pregnant ['pregnənt]　　adj. 怀孕的；孕育着…的；富于想象的；富于成果的

preoccupied [pri'ɔkjupaid]　　adj. 全神贯注的，入神的

prescription [pri'skripʃ(ə)n]　　n. 处方，药方；指示

prior to　　在…之前

priority [prai'ɔrəti]　　n. 优先，优先权；优先考虑的事

psychology [sai'kɒlədʒi]　　n. 心理学；心理状态

pyelonephritis [ˌpaiələʊni'fraitis]　　n. 肾盂肾炎

R

radical ['rædikl]　　adj. 激进的；彻底的；根本的；基本的 n. 激进分子；根基

radioactive [ˌreidiəʊ'æktiv]　　adj. 放射性的

raid [reid]　　v. 劫掠；突击搜捕

range from … to …　　从…到…

rash [ræʃ]　　n. 皮疹

rave [reiv]　　n. 喧闹的宴会；极力赞扬

rectum ['rektəm]　　n. 直肠

recur [ri'kɔː(r)]　　vi. 再发生，复发

recurrent [ri'kʌrənt]　　adj. 再发生的；周期性的

refer [ri'fɜː(r)]　　vt. 使求助于；送交；请教

rehabilitation [ˌriːəˌbili'teiʃn]　　n. 修复；复兴

relieve［rɪ'liːv］ v. 解除，减轻

remedy［'remədi］ n. 补救办法；治疗法

retina［'retɪnə］ n. 视网膜

retinopathy［,retin'ɔpəθi，–'nɔp–］ n. 视网膜病

reversible［ri'vəːsəbl］ adj. 可逆的；可医治的

rheumatic［rʊ'mætɪk］ adj. 风湿病的

rheumatoid［'ruːmətɔɪd］ adj. 患风湿症的；风湿症的

rib［rɪb］ n. 肋骨；排骨

ribbon［'rɪbən］ n. 带；缎带

rotate［rə(ʊ)'teɪt］ vi. &vt. 旋转；循环

<h2 style="text-align:center">S</h2>

saliva［sə'laɪvə］ n. 唾液；涎

sap［sæp］ vt. 使衰竭；使伤元气

scurvy［'skɜːvi］ n. 坏血病 adj. 下贱的；卑鄙的

sebaceous［sɪ'beɪʃəs］ adj. 分泌脂质的；脂肪质的

sebum［'siːbəm］ n. 皮脂

secrete［si'kriːt］ v. 分泌

secretion［sɪ'kriːʃ(ə)n］ n. 分泌；分泌物

sedation［si'deiʃn］ n. 镇静

seedy［'siːdi］ adj. 破烂不堪的；憔悴的

seizure［'siːzə(r)］ n. 突然发作

severity［sɪ'verɪti］ n. 严重；严格；猛烈

shot［ʃɒt］ n. 注射；开枪 v. 注射；射击

slurred［sləːd］ v. 含糊地念

snort［snɔːt］ n. 吸食（毒品）

sodium［'səʊdiəm］ n. <化>钠（Na）

soluble［'sɒljəbl］ adj. ［化］可溶的；可以解决的；可以解释的

spectrum［'spektrəm］ n. 系列；范围

spell［spel］ n. 符咒，咒语

spinach［'spɪnɪtʃ］ n. 菠菜

spontaneous［spɔn'teiniəs］ adj. 自发的，本能的；自然产生的

springy［'sprɪŋi］ adj. 有弹力的

squeeze［skwiːz］ vi. & vt. 挤，捏；压迫

steroid［'stɪərɔɪd；'sterɒɪd］ n. 类固醇；甾族化合物

stethoscope［'steθəskəʊp］ n. 听诊器

stiffness［'stɪfnɪs］ n. 僵硬；坚硬

stimulant ['stimjələnt]　n. 兴奋剂

sting [stɪŋ]　n. &vi&vt. 刺，刺痛

stool [stuːl]　n. 粪便

stroke [strəuk]　n. 中风

subtle ['sʌtl]　adj. 微妙的；巧妙的；敏感的；狡猾的

supplements ['sʌplɪmənts]　n. 增补（物）（supplement 名词复数）

suppository [sə'pozətri]　n. 栓剂

suppressant [sə'presnt]　n. 抑制剂；

suspect [sə'spekt]　vt&vi. . 怀疑

swell [swel]　v. 膨胀；肿胀 adj. 极好的；了不起的；非常棒的

swelling ['swelɪŋ]　n. 肿胀；膨胀

symbolize ['sɪmbəlaɪz]　vi&vt. . 象征

symptom ['sɪm(p)təm]　n. 症状；征兆

syndrome ['sɪndrəum]　n. 综合征

systolic ['sis'tɔlik]　adj. 心脏收缩的

T

tackle ['tæk(ə)l]　vt. 处理

tailor ['teilə]　v. 缝制；调整使适合

tattoo [tæ'tuː]　n. 纹身

tender ['tendə]　adj. 一触即痛的；敏感的

tendon ['tendən]　n. <解>筋；腱

therapy ['θerəpi]　n. 治疗；疗法；疗效；心理治疗；治疗力

thyroid ['θaɪrɔɪd]　n. 甲状腺 adj. 甲状腺的

thyroiditis [ˌθaɪrɔɪ'daɪtɪs]　n. 甲状腺炎

tissue ['tɪʃuː]　n. 薄纸；棉纸；[生] 组织；一套

tonometry [təu'nɔmitri]　n. 眼压测量法

toxins ['tɔksinz]　n. 毒素

transmit [trænz'mɪt]　v. 传输；传播

transparent [træn'spær(ə)nt]　adj. 透明的

transplant [træns'plɑːnt]　vt. 移植；迁移

trap [træp]　n./vt. 陷阱，受限

tremor ['tremə(r)]　n. 战栗，颤抖

trigger ['trigə]　n. 起因 vt. 引发，触发

tumor ['tjuːmə]　n. 肿瘤、肿块

U

undergo [ˌʌndəˈgəʊ]　　vt. 经历；遭受

underlying [ˌʌndəˈlaiiŋ]　　adj. 潜在的，含蓄的

ureter [jʊˈriːtə；ˈjʊərɪtə]　　n. 输尿管

urethra [jʊˈriːθrə]　　n. 尿道

urethritis [ˌjʊrəˈθraɪtɪs]　　n. 尿道炎

urine [ˈjʊərɪn]　　n. 尿

V

vaccine [ˈvæksiːn]　　n. 疫苗

variable [ˈvɛəriəbl]　　adj. 可变的；易变的

variant [ˈveəriənt]　　n. 变量，变异体 adj. 变异的，多样的

vessel [ˈvesl]　　n. 容器；血管

viral [ˈvaɪrəl]　　adj. 病毒的；病毒引起的

vitamin [ˈvɪtəmɪn]　　n. 维生素；维他命

vomit [ˈvɔmit]　　v. 呕吐

vulgaris [ˈvʌlgəris]　　adj. 寻常的

vulnerable [ˈvʌlnərəbl]　　adj. 易受攻击的；易受伤的

W

wheezing [wiːz]　　adj. 气喘

withdrawal [wiðˈdrɔːəl]　　n. 戒断（毒品、酒精等），常与 “症状” 连用，特指医学概念上的 “戒断症状”

wrap [ræp]　　vt. 包；（或包扎、覆盖等）用…包裹

Z

zit [zɪt]　　n. 青春痘；粉刺

Appendix 2 Keys

Unit 1 Asthma

Lead – in

All of the above symptoms are about asthma.

Post reading

A1

1. bronchial tubes narrow   2. fatality rate   3. inhaled asthma triggers   4. cold air

5. certain medications   6. relieve symptoms

A2

1. F   2. T   3. F   4. T   5. F   6. T

B1

1. inflammatory   2. a beta-blocker   3. relieve   4. persistent   5. exacerbations

6. chronic   7. stimuli   8. outgrow

B2

1. d   2. e   3. a   4. b   5. f   6. c

B3

1. characterized   2. lining   3. recurrent   4. chronic   5. bedding   6. stuffed

C1

1. 反复发作的哮喘症状往往导致失眠，白天疲劳，减少活动量，旷工及旷课。

2. 其他诱因可能包括冷空气，极端情绪如愤怒或恐惧，与体育锻炼。

3. 城市化也与哮喘的增加有关，但是这种关系的确切性质尚不清楚。

4. 虽然哮喘不能根治，适当的管理可以控制该病，使人们能够享受高质量的生活。

5. 此外，一些患有轻度哮喘儿童会随着年龄的增长摆脱他们的症状。

6. 持续性症状的人必须长期每日用药，控制潜在的炎症反应，防止症状加重。

C2

1. B   2. D   3. C   4. C   5. C

C3

1. The little girl will outgrow her fear of pet animals.

2. Smiling and laughing has actually been shown to relieve tension and stress.

3. 10, 000 deaths a year from chronic lung disease are attributable to smoking.

4. Stress may act as a trigger for these illnesses.

5. A dentist may decide to extract the tooth to prevent recurrent trouble.

Listening

pet waste smoke wood fumes soaps colds infections weather sudden

Unit 2　Cold and Cough

Lead – in

7，　9，　6，　2，　5，　1，　8，　4，　3

Post reading

A1

1. vomiting　2. 15 – to 30 – milligram　3. accessible　4. disposal　5. track　6. suspicious

A2

1. 过度喝咳嗽药不是青少年的新惯例了。

2. 重要的是父母了解风险并知道如何防止孩子故意过量服用咳嗽和感冒药。

3. 含右美沙芬药物很容易找到，囊中羞涩的青少年也负担得起，完全合法。

4. 右美沙芬的滥用是非常普遍的，根据最近的研究，这种非处方药在商店和在互联网上都很容易买到导致了这个原因。

5. 当消耗量大，右美沙芬也可引起高热，或高热。

B1

1. slurred　2. narcotic　3. antihistamine　4. strapped　5. hyperthermia　6. stockpiling

7. lookout　8. impaired

B2

1. d　2a　3. f　4. c　5. b　6. e

B3

1. chug　2. raid raid　3. intentionally　4. suppressant　5. guzzle　6. vomited

7. impaired

C1

1～5 CACBC　6～10 BBABB　11～15 BDAAB

C2

1～5 ADCBD　6～10 CADBC　11～15 CDBDA　16～20 DCABC

C3

1. She intentionally ignored me and went on working.

2. He looks seedy，for he has been ill for a long time.

3. She had a stomach upset yesterday and vomited several times.

4. Nicotine is a toxic substance.

5. He couldn't lift his impaired arm.

Listening

1. unclog a stuffy nose

2. quiet a cough

3. loosen mucus so you can cough it up

4. stop runny noses and sneezing

5. ease fever, headaches, and minor aches and pains

6. Read labels

7. Taking too much of certain pain relievers

Unit 3　Peptic Disease

Post reading

A1

1. duodenum　2. H. pylori　3. ulceration　4. barium X-ray　5. bleeding　6. antibiotic

A2

1. A peptic ulcer is a break in the inner lining of the esophagus, stomach, or duodenum.

2. The three major causes are H. pylori; NSAIDS; and cigarette smoking.

3. No

4. upper gastrointestinal endoscopy

5. Yes

B1

1. eradicate　2. corrosion　3. digestion　4. develop　5. spontaneous　6. interfere

7. counteract　8. correlate

B2

1. e　2. d　3. g　4. c　5. a　6. h　7. b　8. f

B3

1. initiated　2. variable　3. Acidic　4. neutralize　5. erosion　6. persistent

7. secreted

C1 - 1

1. b　2. a　3. d　4. c

C1 - 2

1. a　2. d　3. b　4. c

C2

1. who　2. which/that　3. which　4. which　5. which/that　6. which/that　7. who

8. which　9. which　10. which/that　11. which　12. who　13. which

C3

1. This acid can corrode iron.

2. Health is correlated with dietary balance.

3. The eruption of volcanoes is spontaneous.

4. Persistent cough may be a symptom of pneumonia.

5. Pneumonia is the complication we most fear.

Listening

1. irritability   2. ulcer   3. painful   4. lens   5. throat   6. endoscope   7. treatment

8. breakfast   9. water   10. anesthesia

Unit 4   Constipation

Post reading

A1

1. F   2. T   3. NG   4. NG   5. T   6. F   7. T   8. F

A2

1. Constipation means hard stools, difficulty passing stools (straining), or a sense of incomplete emptying after a bowel movement.

2. Irritable bowel syndrome

3. The number of bowel movements generally decreases with age.

4. Medically speaking, constipation usually is defined as fewer than three bowel movements per week.

5. Laxatives should be the last resort.

B1

1. alternates   2. stimulants   3. acute   4. frequent   5. irritate   6. tailored

7. accumulated   8. chronic

B2

laxatives,   diarrhea,   tumor,   barium enema,   stimulant,   suppository

B3

1. acute   2. accumulate   3. distinguish   4. irritable   5. infrequent   6. alternate

C1 – 1

1. b)   2. d)   3. a)   4. c)

C1 – 2

1. d)   2. c)   3. b)   4. a)

C2

1. are   2. (will) live   3. would/should have died (or might/could have died)

4. will feel   5. will be   6. could live   7. would you do   8. would have eaten

9. could change/could have changed   10. would you change/would you have changed

11. had known   12. would have looked after

C3

1. Last week Miss Wang had twenty classes and was so tired as to have an acute laryngo-pharyngitis.

2. Work should alternate with relaxation.

3. He suffered from chronic gastritis after a long time of hard work.

4. You had better not drink tea and coffee before going to bed although they are mild stimulants

5. I didn't sleep last night, so I am irritable today.

Listening

1. home；weight 2. obese；slim 3. metabolisms 4. diet 5. remodel；weight

6. germ-free 7. flat；fat

Unit 5   Urinary Tract Infection

Post reading

A1

1. Four. They are two kidneys, two ureters, bladder and urethra.

2. When you have about a cup of urine in your bladder, your brain tells you it's time to find a bathroom.

3. Girls are more likely than boys to get a urinary tract infection.

4. It hurts or stings when you pee.

You can only pee a little bit at a time.

You have to get up many times in the night to pee.

Your pee is cloudy.

It smells bad when you pee.

A2

1. urethritis, cystitis, pyelonephritis；

2. bacteria, the urethra, irritation；

3. the urethra, the bladder, irritation；

4. bacteria, the kidney

B1

1. extracted 2. feverish 3. sting 4. irritation 5. trap 6. chill

B2

1. kidney 2. ureter 3. bladder 4. urethra

B3

脑膜炎； 脊柱炎； 鼻炎

C1

1. B   2. C   3. C   4. C   5. A   6. B   7. B

C2

1. C   2. D   3. B   4. D   5. D

C3

1. His father died, leaving him a lot of money.

2. She was so angry that she threw the toy on the ground, breaking it into pieces.

C4

1. D   2. C   3. C   4. D   5. C   6. B

C5

1. No matter how hard I work, there is always more to do.

2. He dropped the glass, breaking it into pieces.

3. Linda's purse is the same style as Jimmy's.

4. I don't know where to start.

5. Bacteria love to grow in warm, moist feverish places.

Listening

Part A

1. T   2. F   3. T   4. T   5. F

Part B

1. Loss of resistance   the bladder

2. contamination   abstraction   inefficiency

3. wet swimming suits   tight clothing   no longer

4. frequency   urgency   voiding   inability to void   painful urination

5. hydration   elimination   hygiene

Unit 6   Hypertation

Post reading

A1

1. T   2. F   3. F   4. F   5. T   6. T

A2

1. wraps a cuff   2. pushing up against   3. essential, secondary   4. undergo periodic blood pressure screenings   5. tolerance to caffeine

B1

1. persistent   2. essential   3. elevate   4. wrapped   5. undergo   6. guarantee

7. reversible   8. transplant

B2

a – vi, b – i, c – iv, d – ii, e – iii, f – v

B3

高血压，低血压；肾上腺皮质的，皮层（质）自主的

C1

1. D　2. B　3. B　4. C　5. D　6. A

C2

1. B　2. A　3. D　4. D

C3 – 1

1. while at college

2. as soon as possible

3. while expanding the old one

C3 – 2

1. While he was reading the newspaper

2. until you are asked to

3. Once he was a worker

C4

1. When（she was）asked，she didn't answer a word.

2. The more youpractice，the better you can understand.

3. People who work in offices are usually refer to as "white collar workers".

4. There is no guarantee that those who have been selected will be an artist.

5. There appears to be no doubt about it.

Listening

Part A

1. The lecture is about the treatment（the drugs）for hypertension.

2. six major classes.

3. Many hypertension patients can take two or even three of drugs in combination.

4. The speaker encourage you to talk to your doctor about the current research into the effectiveness of these remedies.

5. Local pharmacist.

Part B

1. kidneys，salt，water，decreasing，are paired with，more efficiently

2. artery walls，flow through more easily，pump it hard，goes down

3. blood vessels，the hormone ，constrict

4. Beta-blockers

5. ACE inhibitors，enzyme，coughing

6. prevent，from，dilating，the force of the heart's contraction，less forcefully

Unit 7　Angina

Lead – in

1. A　2. A　3. D　4. D　5. B　6. A

Post reading

A1

1. F　2. F　3. T　4. T　5. F

A2

1. coronary artery disease

2. regular pattern，predicted

3. squeezing，pressure，tightening

4. underlying coronary artery disease，damage to the arteries from other factors，reduced oxygen supply

5. prevent，reduce，relaxing，widening

B1

1. squeeze　2. predict　3. underlying　4. relieve　5. trigger　6. Exposure

7. manifest　8. severity

B2

a. i　b. iv　c. ii　d. v　e. vi　f. iii

B3

atherosclerosis 动脉粥样硬化，athero – 粥样的，

– sclerosis 硬化，dentinal sclerosis：牙质硬化

Anticoagulants 抗凝血剂，anti/ant-against，抗

antibiotics：抗生素，anti-diarrhea action：抗泻作用，anticancer：抗癌

antibody：抗体

C1

1. B　2. C　3. D　4. C　5. C　6. C　7. C

C2

1. A　2. D　3. C　4. B　5. D

C3

1. The glass broken by my son has been swept away.

2. The Town Hall completed in the 1800's was the most distinguished building at that time.

3. We will go to visit the bridge built hundreds of years ago

4. The books written by LuXun are popular

5. Is this the book recommended by the teacher?

C4

1. We will go to visit the bridge built hundreds of years ago.

2. He failed not because he isn't clever but because he didn't work hard.

3. Our school supplies us with a tidy environment.

4. It's dangerous for children to cross the road by themselves.

5. Mistakes due to carelessness may have serious consequences.

Listening

Part A

1. For several years, Arnold has suffered from angina. The symptoms may be pain in the chest or other parts of the body.

2. Because it is a warning of potentially more serious problems.

3. stopping smoking, control your high pressure if you have one, lowering the cholesterol

4. A combination of several angina medications. He takes 14 pills daily.

5. By injecting die

Part B

1. at risk for a heart attack

2. oxygen, nutrient

3. a narrowing of these arteries

4. stress, family history, smoking

5. improve the blood supply to the heart

6. medications

7. inflate it, at gradually increasing pressure, as high as 12 to 14 times

Unit 8   Depression

Conversation

1. C   2. D   3. B   4. A   5. D

Post reading

A1

1. F (group of syndromes)   2. F   3. T   4. T   5. NG

A2

1. Crying spells, body aches, low energy or libido, problems with eating, weight, or sleeping.

2. Because it affects millions of people.

3. Yes.

4. The combination of a major depression and a dysthymia.

5. The answer may vary from person to person.

B1

1. exceed　2. recurred　3. interfere　4. negative　5. encompasses　6. inherit

7. postpone　8. priority

B2

1. d　2. g　3. a　4. e　5. c　6. f　7. h　8. b

B3 – 1

Inter – 表示"在…之间、相互"。1. c　2. a　3. d　4. b

B3 – 2

Dys – 表示"困难"。1. c　2. b　3. a　4. d

C1

1. They threw out the computer that/which ever worked properly.

2. This is the lion that/which has been ill recently.

3. The building which/that is on the other side of the river is an exhibition center.

4. I don't like the man who/that is quarrelling with his colleagues.

5. Have you found the key which/that was lost last week?

C2

1. 濒临语言指的是那些由于科技和文化同化欲求而逐渐消失的语言。

2. 上瘾是一种改变一个人的神经系统的大脑疾病。

3. 人口过剩和淡水短缺是当今人们面临的两大棘手问题。

4. 传统学校提供一些文化和体育活动，这些是在家中接受教育的孩子将会错失的东西。

5. 你昨天在校园里碰到的那些人来自英国。

C3

1. Daily exercise and proper diet is the best way to keep healthy.

2. Please cover the painting with something to prevent it from rain.

3. Someone saw the car which you lost yesterday.

4. The meeting will be taken the form of results show and group discussion.

5. This is the most precious gift that I have received.

Listening

Part A

1. 4，000　2. 1995　3. 5.5；2　4. 7；2002　5. 8

Part B

1. F　2. T　3. F　4. F　5. T

Unit 9　Alcoholism

Post reading

A1

1. F　2. F　3. T　4. F　5. NG

A2

Stages		Features
The First Stage		Be preoccupied with getting intoxicated; develop problems in various aspects of life.
The Second Stage		Having access to alcohol
The Third Stage		Feeling normal only when using alcohol; increased risk-taking behaviors.
The Fourth Stage		Occasional use or regular weekly use of alcohol
The Fifth Stage		Increased frequency, drink on a regular basis

B1

1. minimize　2. hygiene　3. moderation　4. withdrawl　5. vulnerable　6. preoccupied

7. compromise　8. deterioration

B2

1. g　2. d　3. c　4. h　5. b　6. f　7. a　8. e

B3 − 1

− osis 表示"病症"。1. c　2. b　3. d　4. a

B3 − 2

− de 表示"剥离"。1. d　2. b　3. a　4. c

C1

1. 这些装饰品不能互相比较，它们是不同的风格。

2. 今天之前没有人收到过通知。

3. 闲暇时间里，这个男孩不是打篮球就是玩电脑游戏。

4. 我想我会去野外走走而不是呆在家里。

5. 过量饮酒导致他现在的身体状况特别糟糕。

C2

1. simple sentence　2. complex sentence　3. simple sentence　4. simple sentence

5. compound sentence　6. complex sentence　7. compound sentence

8. complex sentence　9. simple sentence　10. simple sentence

C3

1. We should engage in more meaningful and useful things for our society.

2. Obviously, they are paying as much effort as we do.

3. They are suffering from healthy problems and worrying about other problems caused by radiation.

4. The ages of patients suffering from hypertension ranging from teenagers to the old.

5. I know the girl that was taken away by the policeman for drunk driving.

Listening

1. True 2. False 3. False 4. True 5. True 6. False 7. True 8. True

Unit 10　Diabetes

Lead – in

1. B 2. B 3. D 4. B 5. B 6. B 7. D 8. C

Post reading

A1

1. blood glucose (sugar)

2. insulin, pancreas, cells

3. kidneys, nerves

4. three, type 1 diabetes, type 2 diabetes, gestational diabetes

5. adult blindness, end-stage renal disease, gangrene, amputation

6. overweight people, older people, racial group

7. Making healthy food choices, eating right amounts of food, being active everyday, staying at a healthy weight

8. Whole grain foods, non-fat or low fat milk, fresh fruit (fresh vegetables); white bread, whole milk, sweetened fruit drinks (regular soda, potato chips, sweets, desserts)

A2

1. It is stored in the liver and muscles.

2. There are three main types of diabetes.

3. Polydipsia (thirsty), polyuria (frequent urination), polyphagia (hunger), and excessive weight loss.

4. The key to taking care of diabetes is to keep the blood glucose as close to normal as possible.

B1

1. fast 2. impeding 3. juvenile 4. Excessive 5. destabilize 6. prediction

7. onset 8. shot

B2

polyphagia, polydipsia, polyuria;

hyperglycemia, hypoglycemia, pancreas;

Step1：Glucose；Step2：Glucose；Step3：Glucose，insulin；

Step4：Glucose；Step5：Glucose

B3

a. vi　b. v　c. vii　d. ix　e. viii　f. ii　g. iv　h. iii　j. i

B4

排尿困难，心电图，神经疾病，皮下注射，高比重的，病理学，失眠，自我吞噬

C1

1. C　2. B　3. D　4. D　5. A

C2

1. Mary is being interviewed.

2. My car is being repaired.

3. The disease is being studied.

4. Our environment is being polluted.

C3

1. Children are being taken good care of.

2. What experiment is now being done?

3. Yesterday I went shopping, bought some books and was treated a big meal by Tom.

4. What do you think is the key to keeping a sound weight? I think the key is to exercise regularly.

5. The key is to keep the body as close to its normal operating temperature of 37 degrees Celsius as possible.

Listening

Part A

1. F　2. F　3. T　4. F　5. T

Part B

1. diabetes, glucose　2. insulin or hormone　3. satellite dishes, westernized

4. necessarily, physical active　5. manageable, preventable

Unit 11　Hyperthyroidism

Post reading

A1

1. F　2. T　3. F　4. F　5. F

A2

1. makes, releases

2. hormones

3. increased heart rate, increased perspiration and a tendency to become more tired

4. autoimmune，antibodies，tissues

5. hyperfunctioning thyroid nodules，thyroiditis

B1

1. fatigue   2. pounding   3. irritable   4. perspiration   5. bulge   6. subtle   7. inflame

8. blurry

B2

a. iv   b. v   c. iii   d. i   e. ii

B3

甲亢，甲亢，甲减，甲减，甲状腺炎，支气管炎，脑膜炎，扁桃体炎

C1

1. D   2. C   3. C   4. C   5. A

C2

1. for   2. on   3. with   4. at   5. through

C3

1. for whom   2. with which   3. on which   4. during which   5. of whom

C4

1. West Lake which Hangzhou is famous for is a beautiful place.

2. The scientist with whom my father worked went abroad last week.

3. There is a big window in my room through which I can see lovely sea.

4. I lost my glasses without which I could see nothing.

C5

1. She is often mistaken for her twin sister.

2. Bacteria vary greatly in their sensitivity to the antibiotic penicillin.

3. They have a tendency to show off，to dramatize almost every situation.

4. People change their mind for a variety of reasons.

5. A supplement to this dictionary may be published next year.

Listening

Part A

1. F   2. F   3. T   4. F   5. T

Part B

1. over two years   2. weight loss   heat intolerance   3. allergic reaction   4. surgery

5. Artery embolization   6. life-threatening side effects   7. benefit from

Unit 12   Acne

Lead – in

1. Acne is considered a disorder. Acne is typically triggered by hormones within the

body. However, no matter what you hear, Acne is not caused by lack of cleaning yourself. You could be the cleanest person in the world and still probably get acne breakouts. It is more likely that you get Acne from washing or cleaning your skin too much versus too little.

2. Wrong! Acne just does not affect teens. Adult acne is on the rise. It is becoming more common than people would have expected. It seems to be more up to genetics than anything else.

3. Prevention methods are really the same all around; it doesn't matter what type of skin or what form of acne you have. Make sure your skin is clean, you do not pick, scratch, or pop blemishes, avoid oil products, drink a lot of water, and make sure to see a dermatologist.

4. There are many treatment options available for people suffering with all different types of Acne. Over-the-counter products are the most popular. They tend to treat light or moderate outbreaks. Severe acne requires time with a dermatologist. A dermatologist will most likely have to prescribe treatment to severe cases.

5. Everyone's acne is different. For some it may only take a couple days, for others is could take two months. It depends on the type of skin and the severity of the case. Be sure to complete any and all treatment methods completely before thinking about more harsh treatments. It shouldn't matter so much on how long your Acne is going to take to clear up. The fact that it is going to clear up is what is important.

Post reading

A1

1. stages 2. disfigures affects 3. getting acne 4. hormones 5. menstrual cycle
6. severity

A2

1. F 2. T 3. F 4. T 5. T

B1

1. b 2. a 3. d 4. e 5. f 6. c

B2

1. disorder 2. disfigures 3. blocked 4. density 5. heredity

B3

dis - 分开；分离；否定；不

1. dis <u>ability</u>　残疾；无力　　2. dis <u>function</u>　功能障碍

3. dis <u>believe</u>　怀疑；不信　　4. dis <u>like</u>　不喜欢；厌恶

5. dis <u>cover</u>　发现；碰见　　6. dis <u>obey</u>　违反；不服从

C1

1. D 2. A 3. D 4. C 5. D 6. D 7. D 8. A 9. B 10. A

C2

1. dis 2. dis 3. dis 4. il 5. il 6. il 7. im 8. im 9. ir 10. ir 11. in 12. in

13. in 14. in 15. un 16. un 17. un 18. un 19. un 20. un

C3

1. Allocate the food to those who need it most.

2. You can be paid in cash weekly or bycheque monthly; those are the two alternatives.

3. The ceremony was an ordeal for those who had been recently bereaved.

4. Handmade goods appeal to those who are tired of cookie-cutter products.

5. Only those over 70 are eligible for the special payment.

Listening

1. the injection of a steroid   relieve some of the pressure   drain out   acne lesion

2. apply ice   calm down   hurt your ankle

3. tenser   superficial   drain

4. ibuprofen   discomfort

Unit 13   Vitamin Deficiency

Lead-in

1. Vitamins help in keeping our eyes, bones, teeth, and gums healthy.

2. Lack of vitamins in the body can cause deficiency diseases.

Post reading

A1

1. folic acid 2. red blood 3. alcohol 4. increasing 5. four 6. normal

A2

1. The main functions of vitamin B_9 are making and repairing your DNA and producing red blood cells

2. The symptoms of folate deficiency are tiredness, weakness, heart palpitations, shortness of breath, headaches, irritability, and difficulty concentrating.

3. The main effects of folate deficiency are folate deficiency anaemia, neural tube defects and Heart disease.

4. Leafy, green vegetables contain high sources of vitamin B_9.

5. Folate (vitamin B_9) deficiency can be treated by increasing the amount of folate-rich foods you eat or by taking a folic acid supplement.

B1

1. c 2. d 3. e 4. f 5. a 6. b

B2

1. deficiency 2. concentrating 3. anaemia 4. spinal 5. supplement 6. fortified

B3

pre-前，预先   fore-前，先，预告   inter – 在…之间，互相

preselect 预选 forehead 额头 interaction 互动

sub-下，低于，次于   over-过度   de-不，非，使相反

subway 地铁 overtime 加班 degrade 降级

B4

1. 无，不，非 2. 反抗 3. 自动，自己 4. 远 5. 生命，生物 6. 共同 7. 反，对应 8. 回，再，重新 9. 以外，超过 10. 在…上，超

C1

1~5 AADBA 6~10 ABCCA   11~15 AADAD

C2

1. Folate（vitamin B_9）is water – soluble.

2. It has also been fortified with vitamin B_9.

3. I'd like a room whose window looks out over the sea.

4. Nobody knew the reason why he was late for school.

5. Excessive folic acid supplementation may harm your health.

Listening

Part A

1. Scientists have discovered thirteen kinds of vitamins.

2. If we do not get enough of the vitamins we need in our food, we are at risk of developing a number of diseases.

3. Vitamin C is needed for strong bones and teeth, and for healthy blood passages. It also helps wounds heal quickly.

4. The study involved more than six thousand individuals.

5. People who know they lack a vitamin should take vitamin supplements, but taking too much of some vitamins can be harmful.

Part B

1. substances reactions 2. 1912 rice 3. prevent cure 4. Infections blindness 5. nervous weak 6. blood normally

Unit 14 AIDS

Post reading

A1

1. NO 2. YES 3. NO 4. NO 5. YES 6. NG 7. NO 8. NG

A2

1. D 2. H 3. C 4. A 5. F 6. G

B1

1. exposure   2. vulnerable   3. transmission   4. Infectious   5. pregnancy   6. diagnosis

7. available   8. symptoms

B2

a. iii   b. v   c. vi   d. i   e. ii   f. iv

B3

1. 反感   2. 抗细菌的   3. 对立面   4. 同情   5. 综合，结合

6. 同义词   7. 排除，赶出   8. 放出，呼气

C1

1. √   2. enjoyed   3. have already seen   4. have just received   5. were

C2

1. C   2. D   3. D   4. D   5. A

C3

1. This is the best film I have ever seen.

2. It's only since I have been blind that I have begun to see through him.

3. John can do it quite well now because he has tried many times.

4. HIV has spread to every corner of the globe since the virus was first identified,

5. Testing for HIV is a two-step process involving a screening test and a confirmatory test.

Listening

Part A

1. C   2. B   3. D   4. C   5. A

Part B

1. announce the discovery, stop more than ninety percent, protect

2. infectious, attaching to

3. has a chance to enter the cells

4. naturally, Combinations of drugs

5. becoming infected with HIV, preventive, increasingly, hardest-hit

Unit 15   Arthritis

Post reading

A1

1. inflammation   2. osteoarthritis   3. stiffness   4. rheumatologist   5. disability

6 dependent

A2

1. Arthritis is inflammation of one or more joints, which results in pain, swelling, stiffness, and limited movement.

2. Broken bone; infection; an autoimmune disease; general "wear and tear" on joints

3. The bones rub together, causing pain, swelling, and stiffness.

4. When there is fluid collecting around the joint, people may feel painful or difficult to rotate the joints in some directions. This is known as "limited range of motion".

5. The particular cause, joints, severity, how the condition affects your daily activities, age and occupation.

B1

1. low-impact　2. individualize　3. deformed　4. tailor　5. alternative　6. prompt

7. pronounced　8. preferable　9. wear and tear　10. exacerbate

B2

1. B　2. A　3. D　4. B　5. A

C1

1. strong　2. usual　3. regular　4. true　5. bitterly　6. common　7. wonderful　8. heavy

9. genuine

C2

1. A　2. D　3. C　4. C　5. B　6. C　7. D　8. B

C3

1. Arthritis involves the breakdown of cartilage.

2. The joint may be tender when it is gently pressed.

3. It is very important to take your medications as directed by your doctor.

4. Tylenol is first-line treatment for osteoarthritis.

5. Rest is just as important as exercise.

Listening

1. F　2. T　3. T　4. F　5. F　6 T

Unit 16　Cataract

Post reading

A1

1. F　2. F　3. T　4. T　5. F

A2

1. steroid, exposure, diabetes

2. blurring, the cloudy lens, replaced, artificial

3. halo

4. widen, dilate, pupils

5. examinationtreatment, macular, degenerationdiabetic, retinopathy

B1

1. comprehensive   2. interfere   3. transparent   4. artificial   5. blurs   6. dilates

7. fade   8. glare

B2

a – v，b – iv，c – ii，d – i，e – iii

B3

病理学 动物病理学 神经病 水疗法

C1

1. do   2. painted   3. to answer   4. built   5. burning   6. done   7. clean

C2

1. C   2. A

C3

1. shouldn't be allowed   2. Must，be watered   3. Yes，it should   4. should be allowed

5. can plant

C4

1. There is convincing evidence of a link between exposure to sun and skin cancer.

2. Contrary to popular belief，moderate exercise actually decreases your appetite.

3. Running a kitchen involves a great deal of discipline and speed.

4. The teacher referred me to Chapter III.

5. Cataract is usually a result of aging and diabetes.

Listening

Part A

1. F   2. F   3. F   4. T   5. T

Part B

1. magnifying glass   clear and flexible   vision problems

2. a probe

3. the use of the surgery microscope   capsule   cortex   nucleus

4. incision   the chocolate layers

5. regular   implants toric implants   multifocal implants   a pear   bifocal lens

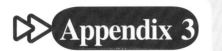 **Appendix 3**   **Listening Scripts**

Unit 1   Asthma

What Causes Asthma?

People with asthma have inflamed airways that are supersensitive to things which do not bother other people. These things are called "triggers." Although asthma "triggers" vary from person to person, some of the most common include:

Substances/Allergens such as dust mites, pollens, moulds, pet dander, and even cockroaches and their waste.

Irritants in the air, including smoke from cigarettes, wood fires or charcoal grills. Also, strong fumes or odors like household sprays, paint, petrol (gasoline), perfume, and scented soaps.

Respiratory infections such as colds, flu, sore throats, and sinus infections. These are the most common asthma triggers in children.

Exercise and other activities that make you breathe harder.

Weather such as dry wind, cold air, or sudden changes in weather.

Unit 2   Cold and Cough

Cold and Cough Medicines

Sneezing, sore throat, a stuffy nose, coughing —— everyone knows the symptoms of the common cold. It is probably the most common illness. In the course of a year, people in the United States suffer 1 billion colds.

What can you do for your cold or cough symptoms? Besides drinking plenty of fluids and getting plenty of rest, you may want to take medicines. There are lots of different cold and cough medicines, and they do different things.

⊙ Nasal decongestants—unclog a stuffy nose

⊙ Cough suppressants—quiet a cough

⊙ Expectorants—loosen mucus so you can cough it up

⊙ Antihistamines—stop runny noses and sneezing

⊙ Pain relievers—ease fever, headaches, and minor aches and pains

Here are some other things to keep in mind about cold and cough medicines. Read labels, because many cold and cough medicines contain the same active ingredients. Taking too much of certain pain relievers can lead to serious injury. Do not give cough medicines to children under four, and don't give aspirin to children. Finally, antibiotics won't help a cold.

Unit 3　Peptic Disease

Patient: Doctor, here is the result.

Doctor: OK. Let me see. The X-ray doctor found irritability and distortion of the duodenum although there was no actual visible ulcer on the X-ray. This does not necessarily mean that you have no ulcer. Let me give you a gastroscopy.

Patient: I heard that it was really painful to have a gastroscopy. How is it done?

Doctor: Don't worry. It will be over soon. I will pass a hollow tube equipped with a lens called endoscope down your throat and into your esophagus, stomach and small intestine. Using the endoscope, I try to look for ulcers.

Patient: Oh, gosh! It's terrible.

Doctor: This is good for your treatment. Don't be afraid. Did you have your breakfast this morning?

Patient: No.

Doctor: How about after 8 o'clock last night?

Patient: No, I had nothing after supper at 6 o'clock, even water.

Doctor: That's fine. Do you need to do it under anesthesia.

Patient: That will make me feel less painful?

Doctor: Yes, just like sleeping. After sleeping, it will be over.

Patient: OK.

Unit 4　Constipation

Our bodies are home to trillions of other organisms that influence our health-and probably our weight.

Researchers found that mice given gut microbes from obese humans became fatter than those that got microbes carried by slim folks.

When the husky and lean mice shared microbes with each other, the bigger ones picked up some of the beneficial gut flora—and had improved metabolisms.

But this shift only occurred if the mice were on a high-fiber, low-saturated fat diet.

If they were on a junk food diet, no improvement.

The findings are in the journal Science.

It's not clear how humans might remodel our microbial communities to change health or weight class.

The mice in the study were raised in germ-free environments and had no native microbiomes of their own.

In people, so-called fecal transplants have been reserved for more severe conditions than a bulging belly.

And probiotic products, such as yogurt, are minimally effective.

But flat or fat, what your belly looks like on the outside might have a lot to do with what's on the inside.

Unit 5 Urinary Tract Infection

Approximately five million people per year seek medical attention for urinary tract infections or UTIs. A urinary tract infection is an inflammation of the urinary tract most commonly caused by Escherichia bacteria, commonly called E-coli.

Normally the bladder has several protective mechanisms that keep the environment sterile despite contamination. Loss of resistance to invading organisms and incomplete emptying of the bladder compromises these protective mechanisms. E-coli gain access to the bladder most often by ascending from the urethra; the organism then attaches itself to the inner lining of the bladder and colonization begins.

For the most part, factors predisposing clients to UTI result in contamination of the tract, obstruction of the tract or inefficiency in the function or structure of the tract. There are several risk factors that increase urinary tract exposure to contaminants and cause urinary stasis, thus providing greater opportunities for the organism growth and survival. Factors that can lead to contamination of the urinary tract include a relatively short urethra in females, insertion of indwelling catheters, straight catheterization, cystoscopy, urethral dilation, sexual intercourse, and menopause related changes. Factors that can lead to obstruction of the urinary tract include renal calculi, commonly called kidney stones, utheralcalculi, and congenital abnormalities. Factors that can lead to inefficiency of urinary tract function and structure include benign prostatic hypertrophy, neurogenic bladder, and anticholinergic medication. Other contributing factors that were once believed to cause UTI, such as tampon use, wet swimming suits, panty hose, and tight clothing are no longer considered significant in the development of UTI.

The reason that so many people seek medical attention for UTI is directly related to the signs and symptoms that develop in response to the inflection. Only about ten percent of clients with UTI are asymptomatic. Most clients that are very symptomatic can report: frequency, urgency, voiding in small amounts, inability to void, inability to empty the bladder, painful urination (called dysuria), cloudy urine, foul-smelling urine, hematuria, lower abdominal discomfort, lower back pain, fever, chills, malaise, nausea, vomiting, and a change in mental status in elderly clients.

A urinalysis can be used as a screening mechanism for clients who have the characteristic symptoms. Typically, the presence of nitrates and WBCs indicate the bacteria are present in the specimen. A urine culture is necessary to confirm the diagnosis of UTI. Colony counts 100, 000 per milliliter have been used in the past to conform UTI. But active infection can exist with much lower colony counts.

Once the diagnosis has been confirmed, antibiotic therapy can be initiated. However, the health care team should investigate the underlying cause of the infection. The presence of symptoms will determine whether or not antibiotics should be prescribed. Symptomatic clients will take antibiotics for three to seven days depending on their age, whether or not they are pregnant and their frequency of infection.

Trimethoprim-sulfamethoxazol——trade name Bactrim, and Nitrofurantoin——trade name——Macrobantin are common first-line choices for treating UTI. Cephalosporins may be used if urine cultures indicate that they are appropriate, and Fluroquinolones——Cipro, for example, may be necessary if the infecting organism is resistant to conventional therapy.

Advise clients to increase their fluid intake to 3 to 4litres per day unless the fluid increase might worsen a coexisting disorder such as congestive heart failure. Increasing fluid intake will dilute the urine, relieve bladder irritation, and prevent or reduce urinary stasis. Very simple changes in hydration, elimination and hygiene can make a huge difference in clients' rate of re-infection. So, in addition to increasing fluid intake, teach clients to urinate frequently and wash the genital area daily, wash before and after sexual relations, and practice safer sex. And for women, avoid deodorant feminine hygiene products, and wipe the perineum from front to back.

Unit 6　Hypertension

For those suffering Stage 1 and Stage 2 hypertension, diet and exercise alone simply aren't enough. Fortunately, there are a number of drugs out on the market that help combat even the most severe hypertension. Today, there are six major classes of drugs: Diuretics, Vasodilators, Alpha and Beta Blockers, Angiotensin-Converting Enzyme Blockers and Calcium Channel Blockers.

Diuretics lower blood pressure by helping the kidneys eliminate salt and water, decreasing flow throughout the body. Some diuretics work to dilate the blood vessels allowing more blood to flow through which in turn brings blood pressure down. Diuretics are often a first-line therapy for many patients and the experts agree when Diuretics appear with another drug, they can help that second drug work more efficiently. Diuretics are excellent first choice for some patients but inappropriate in others such as Diabetes. One important side effect for some Diuretics is the loss of potassium, which can be managed by potassium supplements. This complication is uncommon in standard doses of the drug.

The next type of drug, Vasodilators actually relax the muscles on artery walls, causing them to dilate and allow blood to flow through more easily. As a result, the heart doesn't have to pump as hard and blood pressure goes down. Some Vasodilators work directly on the arterials, or small blood vessels, by an unclear mechanism.

A third type of drug, Alpha-Blockers, also works to relax blood vessels. They block the action of hormones in the body that normally cause the blood vessels to constrict or become narrower. With these hormones suppressed, the vessels are kept open, allowing blood to flow through freely. The most common side effects are dizziness and stuffy nose.

Beta-Blockers are another class of drugs that work primarily by reducing the amount of drugs pumped out of the heart. The result is the lowering of the blood pressure.

Next are medicines that stop the production of the hormone Angiotensin II. These drugs are called ACE Inhibitors. ACE stands for Angiotensin Converting Enzyme. Angiotensin II causes blood vessels to constrict, preventing Angiotensin II from being formed, allowing small blood vessels, called arterials, to enlarge, or dilate, resulting in a lower blood pressure. The most common side effect of ACE inhibitors is coughing. ARBs or Angiotensin Receptor Blockers work in much the same way as the ACE inhibitors do. They also block the action of Angiotensin II, which results in dilating the arterials.

Finally, Calcium Channel Blockers prevent calcium from entering the cells of the heart and blood vessel walls. When calcium enters these cells, it causes the heart to beat harder and blood vessels to narrow. Consequently, reducing the calcium lowers the blood pressure by dilating the blood vessels. It also decreases the force of the heart's contractions; when the heart pumps less forcefully, blood pressure is lowered.

It's important to know that many hypertension patients respond well to two or even three of these drugs taken in combination. Based on your overall health, your doctor will work with you to find out the best drug or drug combination for you. Be sure to immediately report to your doctor any side effect you experience with these drugs. He or she may be able to prescribe another drug combination that is better suited to you.

In your research on hypertension treatments, you may have read about various non-prescription or home remedies like Vitamin C or celery-C. Good scientific evidence shows that a significant lowering of blood pressure from these agents is lacking. Furthermore, some alternative remedies may interfere with prescribed medications. If you are currently using or thinking about using a non-prescription home treatment, we encourage you to talk to your doctor about the current research into the effectiveness of these remedies. Your local pharmacists may also be able to provide you with more information about the types of drugs we discussed here.

Now that you know about the various treatment for hypertension, you want to watch our personal story chapter where you will meet the real doctors and patients who deal with this very common disease every day.

Unit 7   Angina

For a person with angina, the exertion of climbing a flight of stairs can be a frightening hurdle to face. For several years, Arnold York has suffered from angina. The symptom is pain in the chest or other parts of the body, like the shoulders, upper arms or neck. This pain is the result of narrowing of arteries in the heart. It is important that angina be treated because it is a warning of potentially more serious problems.

Dr. Saul Stern: It means that you are at risk for a heart attack. If one of those arteries were to block completely, part of your heart muscle could die, resulting in a heart attack.

The heart is a powerful pump made out of muscle. Like all muscles, it needs oxygen and nutrients. These are supplied to the muscle by the coronary arteries. The pain of angina is caused by a narrowing of these arteries. One cause is the build-up of deposits from the blood that form on the artery walls.

Dr. Stern: That is caused by a few factors which include hypertension or high blood pressure, smoking, high cholesterol, and Diabetes.

Blood flow in the arteries can be reduced without the build-up of deposits. In time of stress or high demand for heart muscle, the arteries can constrict. Smoking is one known cause, but other factors leading to these constrictions are less well understood.

Dr. Stern: We think that stress may play a role in this. Family history may play a role in this, as well as smoking.

Angina can affect people at any age. Some suffer pain only after strenuous activity like a game of squash. Others, like Arnold York experience pain from exertion as limited as climbing a flight of stairs. The danger is that the severity of angina is not related to the amount of pain.

Dr. Stern: In the treatment of angina, what you're trying to do is to improve the blood supply to the heart, so stopping smoking will certainly help. If you have high blood pressure, controlling your high blood pressure again will help. By stopping smoking then, you will help decrease the blockage in the arteries as well as lower your blood pressure, which again affects the blockage in the arteries. Lowering your blood sugar and cholesterol will again help lower the blockage in the arteries, and again help with the decreasing of the severity of the angina. If these factors don't help the angina, then we do have medications.

Dr. Stern talks to the patient: The Nitroglycerin you are taking for your angina···

Nitroglycerin is a common angina medication. It is taken as pills or as a paste that is absorbed through the skin.

Dr. Stern: What Nitroglycerin does is it tries to open up the blood vessels, the coronary arteries that lead to the heart. By opening up the blood vessels, there is more blood, more oxygen to the heart during times of requirement. Therefore the angina attacks are less in severity.

Another group of drugs taken by Arnold York are called BetaBlockers. They affect his heart by slowing it down. This inhibits the force of the muscle contractions, reducing the heart's need for oxygen and lowering blood pressure. Still other drugs called Calcium Blockers work to reduce the constrictions of the arteries in time of stress. Arnold York takes the combination of several angina medications including Nitroglycerin paste.

Arnold York: I take 14 pills daily and Nitro patches in addition.

By following his medication routine and limiting strenuous activities, he is able to live a fairly active life.

Arnold's wife: He can do most of things that he did before.

Arnold: Oh, yeah. Nothing heavy, nothing strenuous.

Wife: That's one reason we moved into a condo so we don't have the outside work to do we can leave the mowing of the grass······

Dr. Stern: Often the medications and the modification of risk factors is not enough. The angina may be so severe, i. e. the amount of exercises required to bring on an angina attack is so little that the patient is incapacitated. If this happens, surgery is often contemplated.

Coronary Bypass Surgery is performed on patients with a number of restricted arteries. For those with fewer blockages, doctors can use a simpler procedure called Angioplasty. This relieves the blockage by fracturing or traumatizing the build-up of deposits in the artery. This is done by breaking it with a small balloon inflated at the narrowing.

George Bliznick has a single serious blockage, and this is his second Angioplasty. The patient is awake for the entire procedure. Doctors feed a probe called a catheter through an artery in the groin and into the heart. By injecting a die, they can identify where the blockage is located. Before performing the Angioplasty, they analyze the blocked artery.

Dr. Leonard Schwartz: The problem is in the wall of the artery. Lipid fat, scar tissue, is forming in the wall of artery and gradually enlarges to obstruct the flow through the artery. What we do is use some way to change by traumatizing that plaque or the wall of the artery containing the plaque in some way change, probably it is fractured.

Through out the procedure, doctors monitor the blood pressure on either side of the blockage. Once they have determined the exact site and the extent of the blockage, they test the small pump that provides the pressure and also the balloon. The two black bands show the ends of the balloon that will be inflated. When they have checked the balloon, it is fed through the artery in the groin and into the heart. The black markers allow them to position the balloon across the blockage in the artery. When the balloon is in position, the doctors carefully begin to inflate it. They do several inflations at gradually increasing pressure. They can use pressure as high as 12 to 14 times atmospheric pressure.

Dr Schwartz: When it begins inflation, there is a constriction what we call an hour class constriction at the points of the stenosis of the narrowing. The rest of the balloon bulges up in a dumbell fashion around it. We watch that area carefully as we can continue to increase pressure. We'd like to see that suddenly disappear, which we call popping the lesion. That's the best result.

Using pictures taken before and after the procedure, Dr. Morris examines the improvement. This is the restricted artery before the Angioplasty. This is the same artery after the balloon inflation. For a patient, there is some discomfort during the procedure. But afterwards, he will recover quickly.

Patient: Some people may say, but I am not, I'm OK.

Arnold York's angina is being successfully treated with medication, reducing risk factors like smoking and taking care to avoid strenuous exertion. He uses extra Nitroglycerin when he has pain or before doing something strenuous. He and his wife lead an active life, pursuing their many interests: painting, model railroading, and building miniature doll houses. He is doing so well that he does net have to visit his cardiologist every six months as before.

Unit 8 Depression

Teens, Television and Depression

A new study suggests that the more teenagers watch television, the more likely they are to develop depressions as young adults. But the extent to which TV may or may not be to blame is a question that the study leaves unanswered.

The researchers used a national long-term survey of adolescent health to investigate the relationship between media use and depression. They based their findings on more than four thousand adolescents who were not depressed when the survey began in nineteen ninety-five.

As part of the survey, the young people were asked how many hours of television or videos they watched daily. They were asked how often they played computer games and listened to the radio.

Media use totaled an average of five and one-half hours a day. More than two hours of that was spent watching TV. Seven years later, in two thousand two, more than seven percent of the young people had signs of depression. The average age at that time was twenty-one.

Brian Primack at the Universtiy of Pittsburgh medical school was the lead author of the *newstudy*. He says every extra hour of television meant an eight percent increase in the chances of developing signs of depression. The researchers say that they did not find any such relationship with the use of other media such as movies, video games or radio. But the study did find that young men were more likely than young women to develop depression given the same amount of media use.

Doctor Primack says the study did not explore if watching TV causes depression. But one possibility, he says, is that it may take time away from activities that could help prevent depression, like sports and socializing. It might also interfere with sleep, he says, and that could have an influence.

The study was just published in the Archives of General Psychiatry. In December, the journal Social Indicators Research published a study of activities that help lead to happy lives. Sociologists fromthe University of Maryland found that people who describe themselves as happy spend less time watching television than unhappy people. The study found that happy people are more likely to be socially active, to read, attend religious services and to vote.

And that's the VOA Special English Health Report, written by Caty Weaver. For archives of our reports, go to voaspecialenglish. com.

Unit 9　Alcoholism

A new study has found that excessive alcohol drinking costs Americans more than ＄220 billion dollars a year, that amount is equal to almost ＄2 a drink. But study organizers believe the biggest costs come from a loss of worker productivity. Robert Brewer works for America's Centers for Disease Control and Prevention, a public health agency. He helped to produce a report on the study.

The researchers used findings from 2006 to examine different costs linked to heavy drinking. They looked at results from around the United States and found a lot of variation in different parts of the country.

Alcohol-related costs include health care, the cost of trying cases for drinking-related crimes, and property damage from road accidents.

Robert Brewer says the biggest cost is lost productivity. Many people with a drinking problem have lower-paying jobs. He says they may also be less productive when they are at work. "In addition to that, a number of people die of alcohol-attributable conditions. And many of those folks die in the prime of their life. So there's the personal tragedy there. But there's also a huge economic cost to somebody dying, for example, in an alcohol-related motor vehicle crash at age 35. "

The researchers were mainly concerned about the cost of heavy alcohol use. The study didn't look at the effect on individuals who drink a glass of beer or wine with dinner. Mr Brewer says the largest costs come from binge drinking when people drink a lot of alcohol in a short period of time.

The study was based on the economic costs of heavy drinking in the United States, but Mr. Brewer says many nations have problems with what the World Health Organization calls "harmful use of alcohol" "But I think that it is very reasonable to assume that harmful alcohol use is going to result in some of the same consequences in other countries, even if the costs associated with those consequences are different".

The study on the economic costs of excessive alcohol use was published in the American Journal of Preventive Medicine.

Two years ago, a British medical examiner ruled that singer Amy Winehouse died as a result of drinking too much alcohol. Winehouse was only 27 years old. Tests show that she died after drinking too much alcohol. Winehouse was only 27 years old. Tests show that she died after drinking enough alcohol to put her blood alcohol level at more than five times the legal drunk-driving limit. The award winning singer had a well documented battle with drugs and alcohol.

And that's the Health Report from VOA Learning English. Go to our website learningenglish. voanews com to leave comments on our reports and to find more stories for people learning American English. I'm Christopher Cruise.

Unit 10　Diabetes

This is the VOA Special English Health Report.

Today is World Diabetes Day, part of acampaign to urge governments to do more to fight the disease. Organizers warn of a diabetes epidemic affecting two hundred forty-six million people worldwide.

Last December the United Nations passed are resolution to observe World Diabetes Day every November fourteenth. The International Diabetes Federation and the World Health Organization began the event in 1991. The federation is an alliance of diabetes groups. It also has partnerships with drug companies.

People withdiabetes have too much glucose, or sugar, in their blood. The body changes food into glucose for energy with the help of insulin, a hormone. In diabetics, the body produces little or no insulin or has trouble using the insulin that is produced.

As a result, too much glucose remains in the blood instead of entering cells. Over time, the disease can cause blindness, kidney disease and nerve damage. It also can lead to strokes and heart disease.

People with type onediabetes need insulin injections. Many with type two do not. Instead, it can be controlled through diet, exercise and treatment. And people may be able to prevent it.

This year's World Diabetes Daycampaign is about children and adolescents. One of the organizers is Doctor Francine Kaufman. She traveled around the world for a film called "Diabetes: A Global Epidemic." The Discovery Health Channel will show it on Sunday.

Type Ⅱ diabetes used to appear mostly in adults, but now more and more children have it. Doctor Kaufman says it is spreading as more people rise out of poverty in developing countries—— for example, India.

FRANCINE KAUFMAN: "They're in cars all day long, and they've got satellite dishes outside their houses. They are eating more food, and more westernized food and getting overweight and developing diabetes. "

She says another place wherediabetes is spreading is South Africa.

FRANCINE KAUFMAN: "We were in the townships and people were overweight. There is more food available than has been in the past. And people are getting on buses and going to offices and not necessarily being as physically active as they have been in the past. "

Doctor Kaufman says solutions must be developed country by country and patient by patient. In Brazil, for example, a health clinic holds dances to get diabetes patients more active. Doctor Kaufman says the message of World Diabetes Day is that the disease is manageable and, in the case of type two diabetes, preventable.

And that's the VOA Special English Health Report. I'm Barbara Klein.

Unit 11　Hyperthyroidism

Doctor: Any pain?

Stella: No. No more.

Doctor: Ok, do you feel much better?

Stella: I do. Thank you.

54 year old Stella is from California. She has been suffering from Graves Disease for over two years. The symptoms include weight loss, heat intolerance, palpatation and thryroid enlargement. In her battle against illness, Stella visited many doctors around the US. However, due to her rare allergic reaction to some medicines, Stella was told that doctors could not do anything to help her.

Stella: No. I never expected to travel especially this far to get any kind of help. I thought America would be able to help me. I was surprised that they cannot help me.

Thanks to an article published in *The Journal of Clinical Endocrinology Metabolism*, Stella found out about Professor Xiao Haipeng, an author and deputy director of the First Affiliated Hospital of Sun Yat-sen University in Guangzhou.

XiaoHaipeng: She is allergic to all anti-thyroid drugs and she is also allergic to Beta Blockers. Since hyperthyroidism is not well controlled, so surgery is very contraindicated. So we use the embolization therapy to embolize 2 or 3 fine arteries.

Artery embolization is a minimally basic surgery which has been done in China for over ten years. It has been estimated about forty people have been cured in Guangzhou with this method. With a small cut on the left artery, the patient has some of his or her vasculars embolized to partially cut off the blood supply to the thyroid. It's a much safer procedure compared with traditional surgery without life-threatening side effects.

Stella has now recovered from the procedure and is thinking of promoting this new therapy when she returns to the US. She is confident that more patients could benefit from this international exchange of medical expertise.

Unit 12　Acne

How to Deal With Acne Pain

People who have acne know that acne isn't just a cosmetic condition; sometimes the lesions of acne are literally painful. This is caused when you tend to have a deeper acne lesion that can't come to a head and drain. So what do you do to get rid of the pain associated with acne? Well the best choice is to come to a dermatologist.

One, you should be under acne treatment, but if you're still getting these painful lesions, there are things that can be done to alleviate the pain immediately. A popular treatment is the injection of a steroid, which calms down the inflammation. Also, the hole that's made during the injection can also relieve some of the pressure because some of the pus and the keratin plug that is causing the acne and inflammation can drain out. Sometimes a larger needle is used to drain the lesion, because that's the primary way you're going to treat the acne lesion.

If you're at home and you can't get to a doctor, some things that you can do to help with these deep, painful lesions are: if it's early, the lesion is about to form, you can apply ice to the area for a few minutes to calm down the inflammation, much like you'd do if you hurt your ankle doing a sport.

If the lesion is tenser and it looks like it's starting to come to a head and it's more superficial, apply heat may help, like you might do with a boil, to get it to come to a head and drain.

Sometimes taking ibuprofen at home, if that's something that you're able to do and that's safe for you, can help with some of the discomfort of an acne lesion.

But ultimately it's a surgical problem to deal with the pain of an acne lesion, so the best option is to letyour doctor help you with that.

Unit 13　**Vitamin Deficiency**

Vitamins are Important to Good Health

Many jobs must be done with two people. One person takes the lead. The other helps. It is this cooperation that brings success.

So it is with the human body. Much of our good health depends on the cooperation between substances. When they work together, chemical reactions take place smoothly. Body systems are kept in balance.

Some of the most important helpers in the job of good health are the substances we call vitamins.

The word "vitamin" dates back to Polish scientist Casimir Funk in 1912. He was studying a substance in the hull that covers rice. This substance was believed to cure a disorder called beriberi.

Funk believed the substance belonged to a group of chemicals known as amines. He added the Latin word "vita," meaning life. So he called the substance a "vitamin" ——an amine necessary for life.

Funk was not able to separate the anti-beriberi substance from the rice hulls. It was later shown to be thiamine. Other studies found that not all vitamins were amines. So the name was shortened to vitamin. But Funk was correct in recognizing their importance.

Scientists have discovered thirteen kinds of vitamins. They are known as vitamins A, the B group, C, D, E and K. Scientists say vitamins help to carry out chemical changes within cells. If we do not get enough of the vitamins we need in our food, we are at risk of developing a number of diseases.

This brings us back to Casimir Funk. His studies of rice were part of a long search for foods that could cure disease.

One of the first people involved in that search was James Lind of Scotland. In the 1740s, Lind was a doctor for the British Navy. He was investigating a problem that had existed in the Navy for many years.

The problem was the disease scurvy. So many sailors had scurvy that the Navy's fighting strength was very low. The sailors were weak from bleeding inside their bodies. Even the smallest wound would not heal. Doctor Lind thought the sailors were getting sick because they failed to eat some kinds of foods when they were at sea for many months.

Doctor Lind separated 12 sailors who had scurvy into two groups. He gave each group different foods to eat. One group got oranges and lemons. The other did not. The men who ate the fruit began to improve within seven days. The other men got weaker. Doctor Lind was correct. Eating citrus fruits prevents scurvy.

Other doctors looked for foods to cure the diseases rickets and pellagra. They did not yet understand that they were seeing the problem from the opposite direction. That is, it is better to eat vitamin-rich foods to prevent disease instead of eating them to cure a disease after it has developed.

Which foods should be eaten to keep us healthy? Let us look at some important vitamins for these answers.

Vitamin A helps prevent skin and other tissues from becoming dry. It is also needed to make a light-sensitive substance in the eyes. People who do not get enough vitamin A cannot see well in darkness. They may develop a condition that dries the eyes. This can result in infections and lead to blindness.

Vitamin A is found in fish liver oil. It also is in the yellow part of eggs. Sweet potatoes, carrots and other darkly colored fruits and vegetables contain substances that the body can change into vitamin A.

Vitamin B-one is also called thiamine. Thiamine changes starchy foods into energy. It also helps the heart and nervous system work smoothly. Without it, we would be weak and would not grow. We also might develop beriberi.

Vitamin C is needed for strong bones and teeth, and for healthy blood passages. It also helps wounds heal quickly. The body stores little vitamin C. So we must get it every day in foods such as citrus fruits, tomatoes and uncooked cabbage.

Vitamin D increases levels of the element calcium in the blood. Calcium is needed for nerve and muscle cells to work normally. It also is needed to build strong bones.

The medical experts agreed with doctors who say that people who know they lack a vitamin should take vitamin supplements. Some older adults, for example, may not have enough vitamin B-twelve. That is because, as people get older, the body loses its ability to take it from foods.

The experts also noted that taking too much of some vitamins can be harmful. They said people should be sure to discuss what vitamins they take with their doctors.

Several studies have not been able to show that taking vitamin supplements in addition to a balanced diet helps to prevent disease. One study found that older Americans do not get enough Vitamin C and required minerals. The study involved more than six thousand individuals. More than half of them took vitamin supplements.

Vitamins are important to our health. A lack of required vitamins can lead to health problems.

Different vitamins are found in different foods —— grains, vegetables and fruits, fish and meat, eggs and milk products. And even foods that contain the same vitamins may have them in different amounts. Experts say this is why it is important to eat a mixture of foods every day, to get enough of the vitamins our bodies need.

This SCIENCE IN THE NEWS program was written by Brianna Blake.

Unit 14   AIDS

Researchers, policy makers and activists are busy preparing for the International AIDS Conference. The next conference begins Sunday in Vienna, Austria. On Tuesday, the Obama administration announced its National HIV/AIDS Strategy. The plan aims to reduce new HIV infections by twenty-five percent within five years. It also aims to make sure infected patients get treatment more quickly. HIV is the virus that causes AIDS. The government says sixty-five percent of Americans who discover they are infected get treatment within three months. The new plan calls for increasing that to eighty-five percent. Thirty million dollars from the health care reform law is to go to support prevention activities, including expanded HIV testing. Over one million Americans are living with the virus, out of an estimated thirty-three million people worldwide.

Last week, government scientists in the United States announced the discovery of two antibodies that raise hopes for an AIDS vaccine. They say these antibodies can stop more than ninety percent of all known strains of HIV. Antibodies are proteins that the body makes to help protect itself against infection. Researchers made the discovery at the National Institute of Allergy and Infectious Diseases. The director of its Vaccine Research Center, Gary Nabel, says each antibody blocks the virus from attaching to white blood cells.

GARY NABLE: "It reacts with that region, it inactivates the virus and the virus never has a chance to enter the cells that it would otherwise infect."

The antibodies were discovered in a man, known as Donor 45, whose body produced them naturally.

Patients with HIV must take medicine all their lives to prevent AIDS. Combinations of drugs are able to suppress the deadly virus in the body——not a cure in the traditional sense, but the next best thing.

In another development, the United Nations reported Tuesday that the number of young people becoming infected with HIV in Africa is falling.

The U. N. AIDS agency gives credit to better use of preventive measures. It says young people in Africa are waiting longer to have sex. They are also having fewer sexual partners. And they are increasingly using condoms. As a result, the agency says HIV rates are falling in sixteen of the twenty-five hardest-hit countries in Africa.

And that is the VOA Special English Health Report, written by Mario Ritter. I'm Steve Ember.

Unit 15　Arthritis

Finding New Ways to Treat Rheumatoid Arthritis

Rheumatoid arthritis is a painful disease that can destroy joints. Women are three times more likely to get it than men. Rheumatoid arthritis is considered an autoimmune disease, a disease where the body attacks healthy cells. The exact cause is unknown. But in a recent study, an experimental drug showed signs of halting the disorder in laboratory mice.

Harris Perlman is a medical researcher at Northwestern University in Illinois. He says normally a protein in healthy immune cells causes the cells to die after they attack an invading virus or bacteria. But in rheumatoid arthritis, that protein is missing in some immune cells. Instead, the protein builds up in the joints and attacks cartilage and bone.

Professor Perlman developed what he calls a suicide molecule. It acts like the protein that directs cells to self-destruct. He says the suicide molecule halted and even reduced rheumatoid arthritis in seventy-five percent of the mice in the study. He believes the treatment could also work in people.

Current treatments for rheumatoid arthritis can reduce pain, but they do not work for everyone. They also have side effects such as an increased risk of infection. Harris Perlman says the new treatment produced no major side effects in the mice.

The study appeared earlier this year in the journal Arthritis and Rheumatism.

Arthritis is not a single disease. The MedlinePlus Medical Encyclopedia, a United States government website, says there are more than one hundred different kinds.

Arthritis produces pain, swelling and limited movement in one or more joints. It involves the breakdown of cartilage. Joints need cartilage for smooth movement and to absorb shock when you put pressure on a joint.

Arthritis can be caused by injury, infection, an autoimmune disease or just long-term use. Some forms are curable, others are not. Some autoimmune forms of arthritis, if not treated, may cause joints to become deformed.

The most common form of arthritis, osteoarthritis, is more likely to affect older people. It most commonly affects the hips, knees or fingers. Overweight people have a higher risk of osteoarthritis. Other risk factors are repeatedly putting stress on a joint or having an earlier injury.

A physical therapist can design an individualized exercise program to reduce arthritis pain and support healthy joints. Getting plenty of sleep, reducing stress and eating a diet high in vitamins and minerals can also help.

And that's the VOA Special English Health Report. I'm Bob Doughty.

Unit 16　Cataract

This is a topic I find very interesting, so let's see how I do it. I usually talk about this with a lot of patients, so it's very rare I get to give this to health care professionals. So let's talk about cataracts. If we talk about cataracts, we need to define our term. What exactly is a cataract? Well, let's take an eye model and see more videos.

Take an eye model, open it up and look inside, we all have a little magnifying glass inside there, called the lens. The lens is clear and flexible like a gummy bear, and it can change shape and helps us do a lot of fine focusing. Now if that lens becomes cloudy from the ravages of time and ultraviolet light and build up of insoluble proteins inside the eye, then this is what we call a cataract. So a cataract is a lens that becomes cloudy, and that cloudy lens causes vision problems. For most people, the first symptom is night driving, glare, car head-lights and things like that.

A bunch of British fighter pilots had their spitfire cockpit fittings explode on them, ending up getting shrapnel inside the eye, and this shrapnel floated in there and stayed in there for years. And the British ophthalmologists were amazed because this plastic did not become infec-ted, the eyes did not become inflamed. It stayed in there inert, and they came up with the i-dea that maybe, just maybe, we could take a cataract out of the eye, we could make a lens out of Plexiglas, put it back into the eye, and restore vision that way. And that's how modern cataract surgery first started.

And that's exactly what they did. They would take the eye, dilate the pupil very big, make a huge incision, take a cold probe, stick it to that cataract lens so it sticks to it, break the strings, pull the entire cataract out in one giant piece. And then the question is: where do you put the giant piece of Plexiglas? There are not a lot of support structures in the eye. So first of all, they said, let's try the front of the eye, but it rubbed on the cornea, and eventually, you needed corneal transplant surgery. Then they attached nylon strings to the lens and suspen-ded it behind the eye, to compensate, but nylon breaks down over decades and the piece of plastic floated behind the eye. It was just not a good situation, so this was the state until the seventies or so.

Modern surgery really began because of two discoveries. One was the use of the surgical microscope. In the prerious, the surgeries was done with magnified lens loops such as this man is heralding. So the surgical microscope was the first thing that was required.

And the second thing was the discovery of the lens. That that cloudy cataract is not a sin-gle piece, it is not a single piece of glass or plastic or tissue. It's more like peanut M&M in the sense that just like a peanut M &M has 3 layers.

There's a hard candy shell, a chocolate layer, and a peanut in the middle. Now it's these 3 layers that help us change our surgical technique. In fact, if you look at someone who has a really bad cataract, This cataract has gotten so bad, the chocolate layer turned into milk choco-late and kind of milky and watery, and the peanut has gotten so dense and heavy, it's actually sunken into the bottom parts of the candy shell, which is kind of like a zip lock bag. It's clear, so you can't really see it that well.

So, 3 layers! These 3 layers we don't call the candy shell, we call it the capsule on the outside and the nucleus is the peanut in the middle and the cortex is that part in be-tween. These 3 layers have changed how our cataract surgery's done today. We make a very small incision, and we take a little bit of a circle off the hard candy shell in the front. We make a hole in the capsule so we can get access to the inner part of the cataract. Then we take a device called a PHACAEMULSIFICATION unit that vibrates at a very high frequency and breaks up the chocolate layers and breaks up the peanut into very small parts and allows us to vacuum those out through that very, very small incision so we've gotten all of the peanut out, but there's still some chocolate in there; there's still some cortex. Let's remove that cortex, and we end up with the hard candy shell capsule which is like a basket now with a hole in the front.

So there are some new technologies out there now that you've probably heard of. One of these technologies is one that fixes ASTIGMATISM. Now, has anyone been told her they have an ASTIGMATISM? It's very common. We all have a bit of ASTIGMATISM.

So, what is it? Well, the surface of the cornea is supposed to be perfectly round like a basketball-the same axes in every meridian, but with ASTIGMATISM, the surface of the eye is more like a football, so steeper one way and a little bit shallower another way. And because it has 2 axes, it almost has 2 focal points.

Now, what if you have a cataract surgery on Astigmatism? What can we do? Well, there is now an implant that will fix it. Basically, they created that football into the implant itself, and when you put it in the eye, we put it in and then we spin it till it perfectly balances out the cornea's ASTIGMATISM. These are calledToric Implants. They are awesome! As far as I'm concerned, there's no real downside to them other than costing a little bit more because they really decrease the need for glasses for people who have got ASTIGMATISM. It's a really predictable way to fix ASTIGMATISM.

Can there be any downside? Sure, this thing can rotate, and if it rotates in 5 - 10 degrees, then you lose something of the effect you are going for. But my experience is they work very well, and I have compunction about putting this lens in my own eye.

Now, there is another lens that's probably a little bit more exotic and is probably getting a bit more press and is something people use more, and that's Multi Focal implants. You've heard of Restore Lens. Well, here's the problem: we have yet to come up with a lens implant as good as our natural lens. Like I've already said, the lens can change shape like a gummy bear, and it's that thickening and flattening that gives us our focus of a wide range. When we hit about age 40, our ability to change shape of the lens begins to harden, and that hardening of the natural lens of the eye, is a sort of pre-cataract. That makes us have to wear reading glasses because we can't get it round enough. We just can't get it to round out to read, and so we need a little bit of extra help with "cheaters" (reading glasses).

And one of the things we can do is go to the sea because there is a wide variety of eyes out there in the animal kingdom. Especially with the invertebrates. I mean, there's compound eyes, there's mirrors for lenses. There's lots of things. In fact, if we look a fish, like this Little Nimo here, fish are kind of interesting because they've got rock hard lenses inside.

This is an interesting cartoon of a fish I drew last week. It's called an "anablep" otherwise known as the 4 – eyed fish down in South America. And it has very odd looking eyes. It almost looks like it has 2 irises or 2 pupils. It's called the 4 eyed fish for a reason. This fish is neat because it floats on the water with half of its eye above the water and the other half of the eye under the water. And it's able to see predators coming from above and see its food down below. It can do very different things. This is a pretty amazing feat. You see, I wonder, how does it do that? And the way it does it is because the lens in this eye of this fish looks like a pear. It is actually, think about it for a moment, this is almost like a bifocal in glasses. This fish has a bifocal lens inside the eye which allows it to see on top, things up in the air, and things close up under water, through different parts of this lens.

So, today, in modern life, we have 3 choices, roughly, as far as the implants that we use. Regular implants I probably put in 95% of my patients-tried and tested, very good! At the other end of the spectrum, you have these multifocals which have some downsides-haloes, night time vision, but can give a better range of focus. And somewhere in the middle are these Toric Implants that can rectify an ASTIGMATISM, and if you have an ASTIGMATISM, a wonderful implant. Not much downside to it.

References

［1］赵颖，杨晓华．医学英语听说教程［M］．北京：人民卫生出版社，2013.

［2］王小丽．医学英语教程［M］．西安：西安交通大学出版社，2010.

［3］林韶蓉．VOA 医学英语听力教程—健康报道专题［M］．北京：高等教育出版社，2012.

［4］DIANA HOPKINS & PAULINE CULLEN. Grammar for IELTS with answers ［M］．西安：西安交通大学出版社，2013.

［5］侯局左．医药专业基础英语［M］．北京：化学工业出版社，2009.

［6］陈颖君．药学情景英语［M］．北京：中国医药科技出版社，2007.

［7］王玉章，等．译．霍恩比．著．牛津高阶英汉双解词典．7 版．北京：商务印书馆，2009.

［8］Anderson, Douglas M. , et al. Mosby's Medical, Nursing, and Allied Health Dictionary, 6th edition. St. Louis, MO: Mosby. 2003.

［9］Worthington-Roberts, B. , and Williams, S. Nutrition in Pregnancy and Lactation, 6th edition. Madison, WI: Brown and Benchmark, 1997.

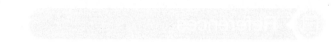